The Gynecological Papyrus Kahun

Authored by Helena Trindade Lopes
and Ronaldo G. Gurgel Pereira

Published in London, United Kingdom

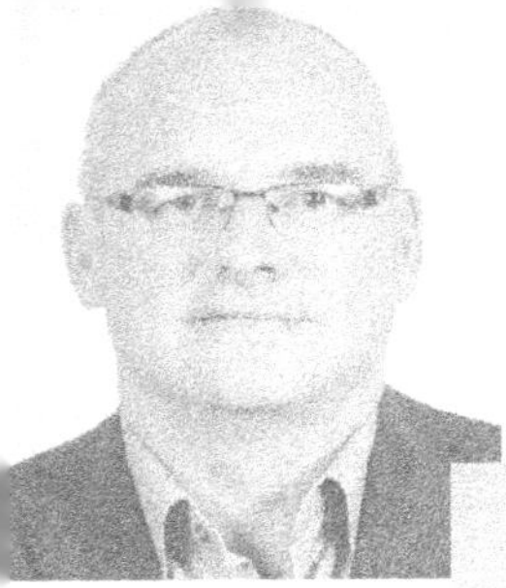
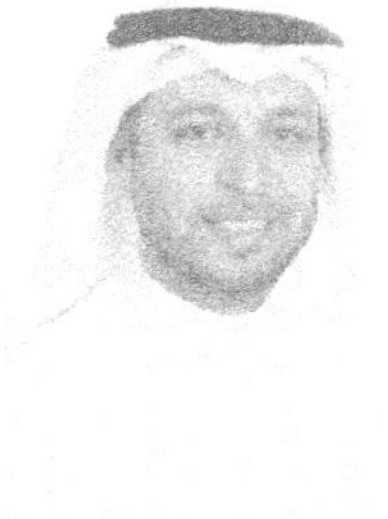
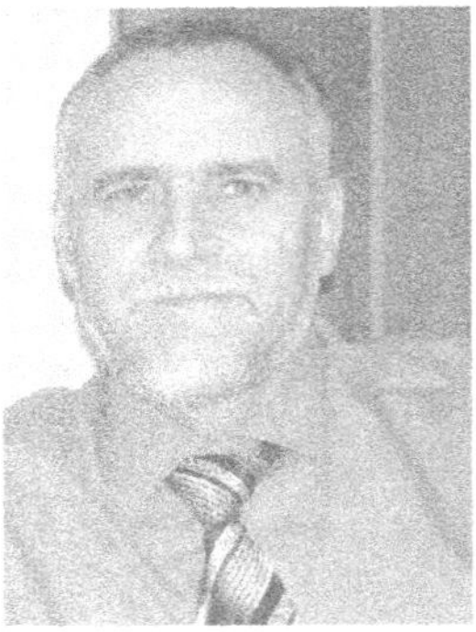
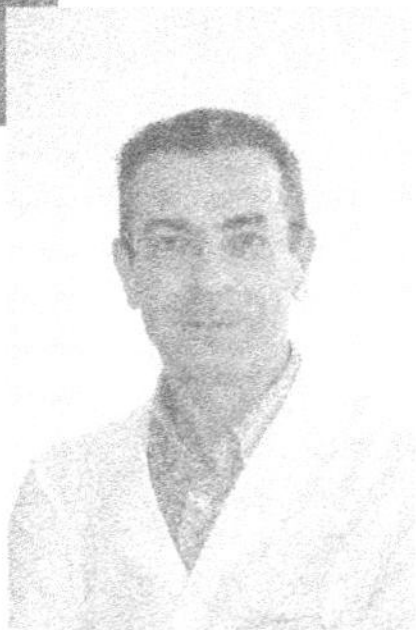
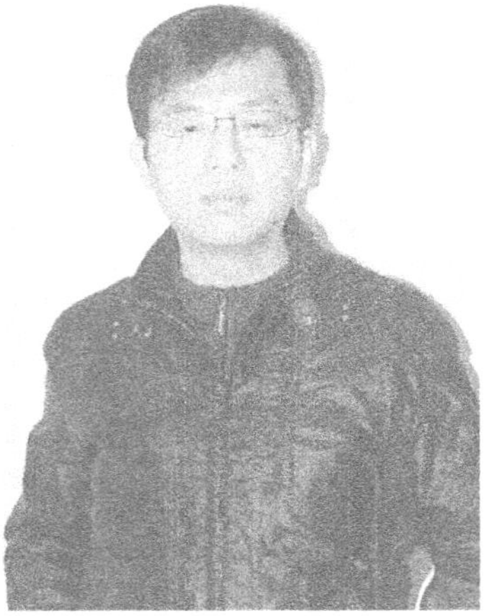
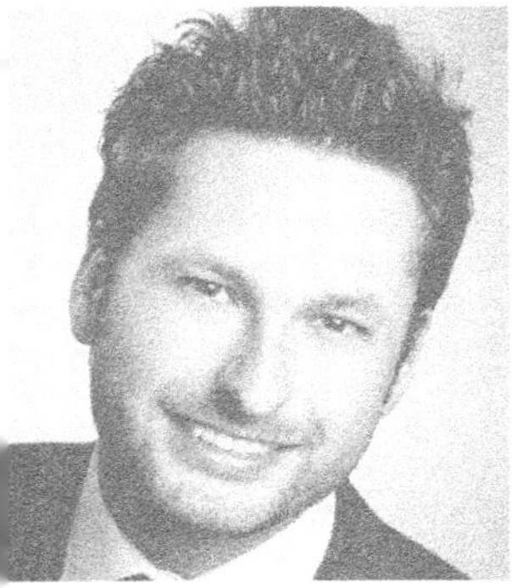
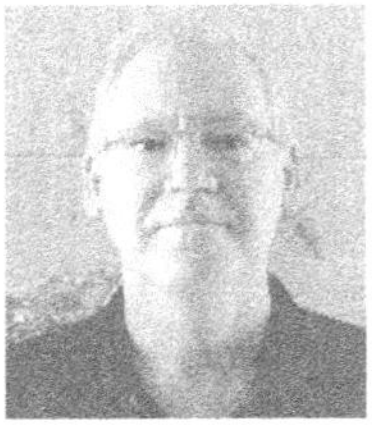

IntechOpen

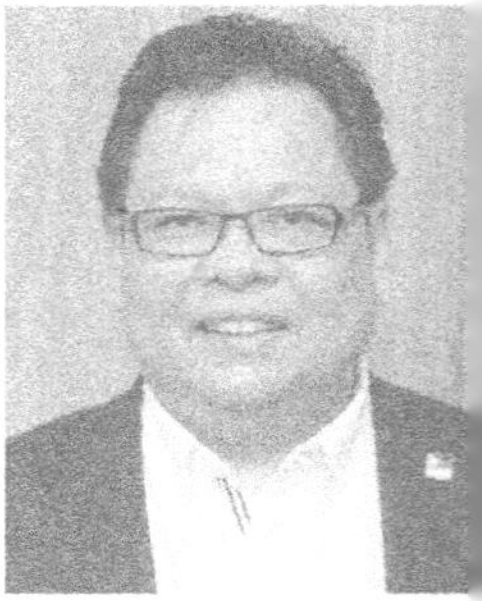
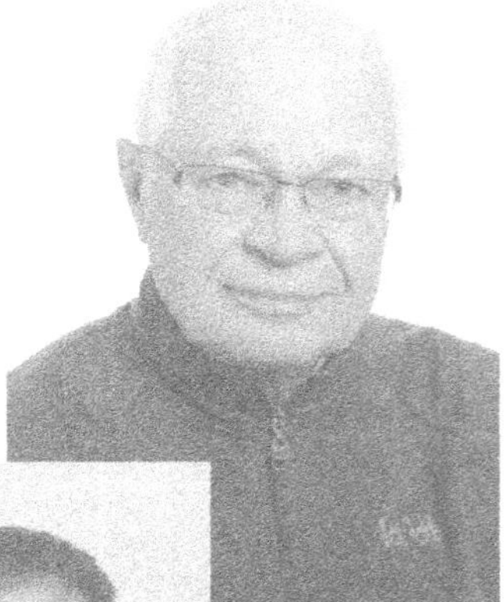
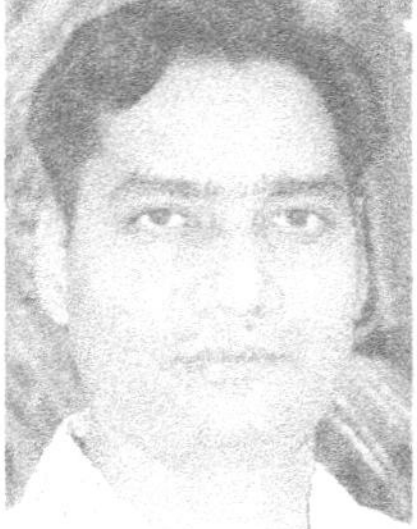
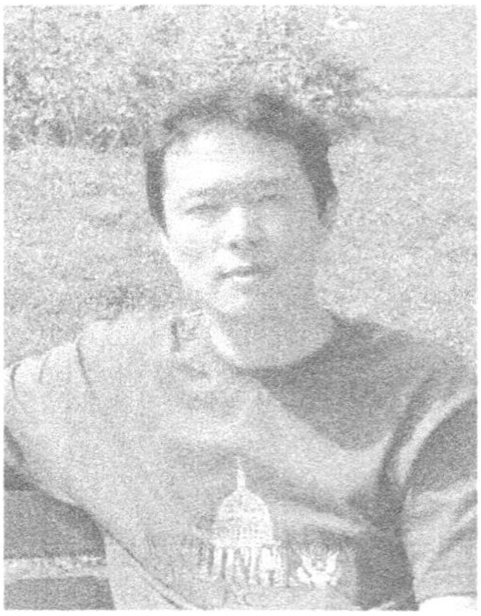
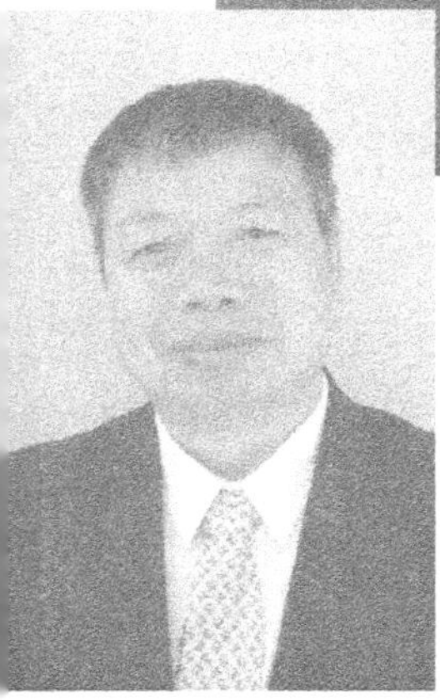
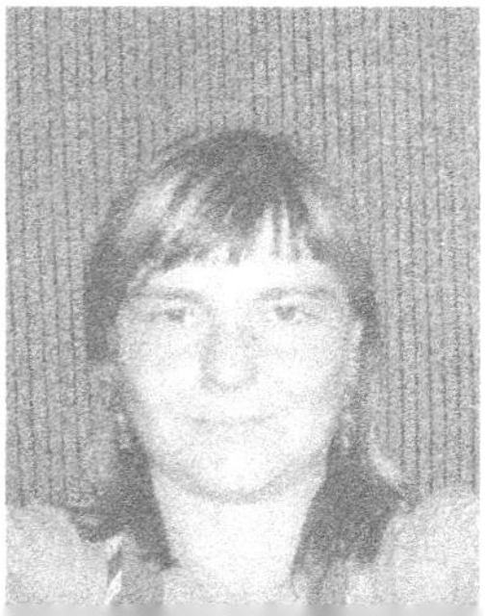

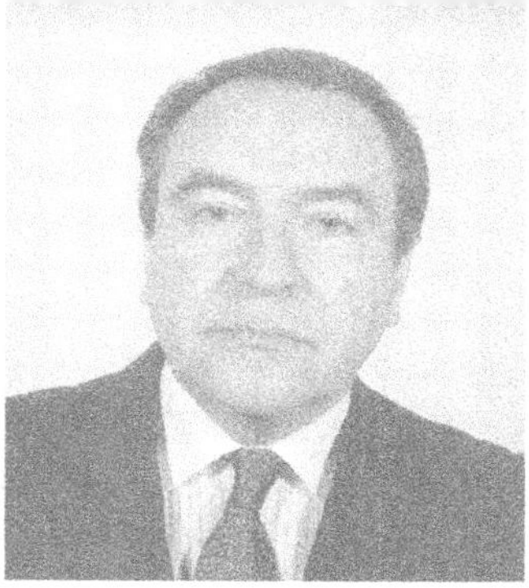
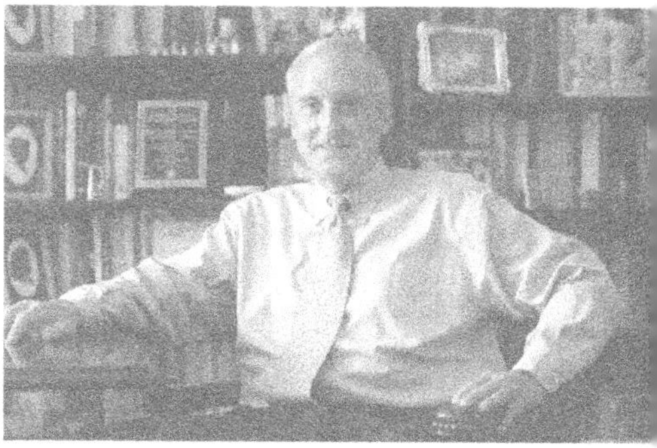
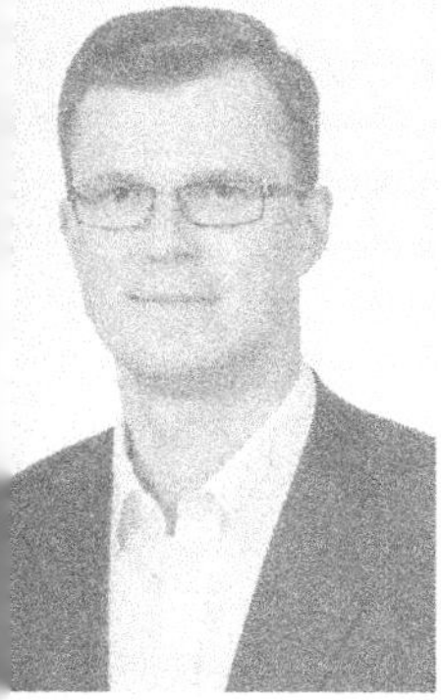
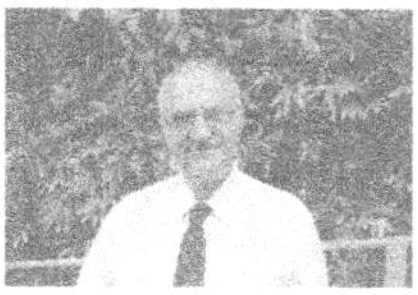
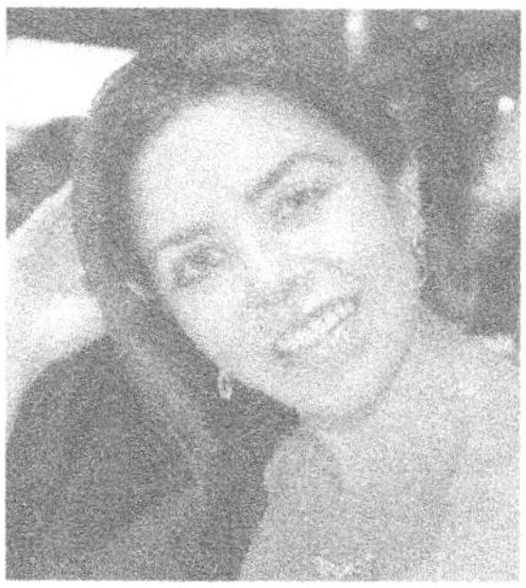

Supporting open minds since 2005

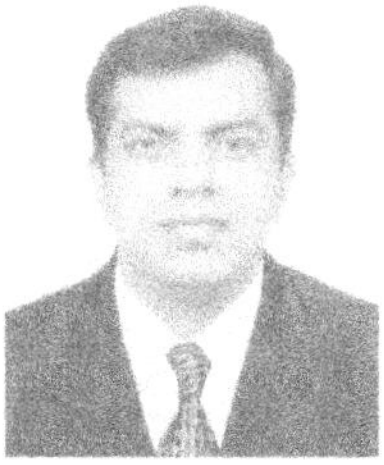
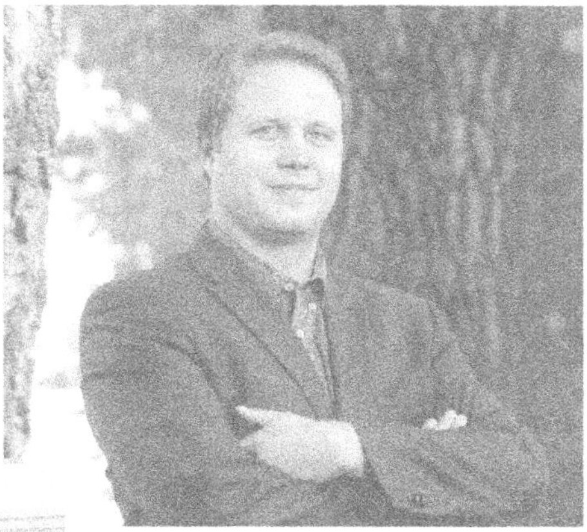
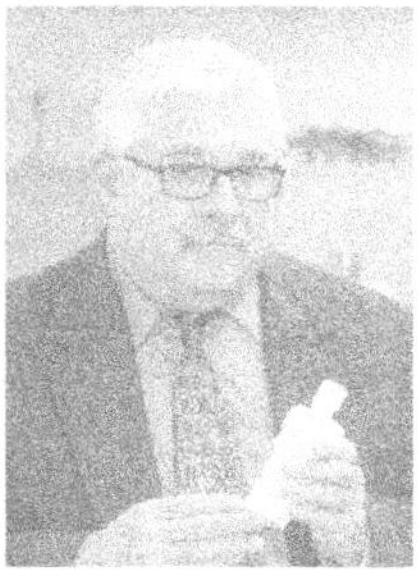
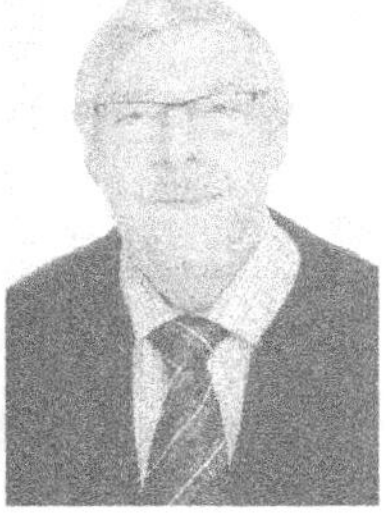
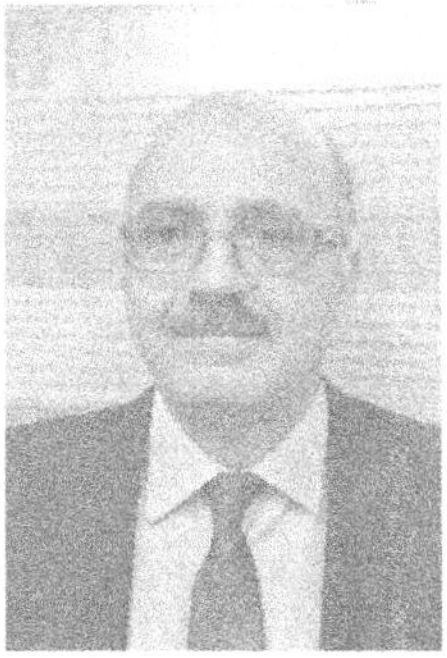
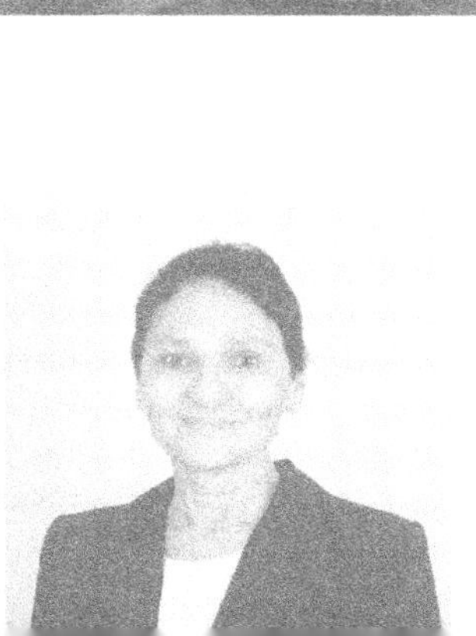
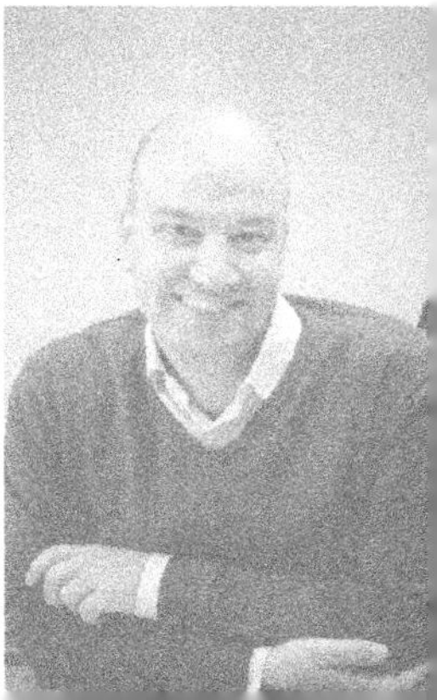

The Gynecological Papyrus Kahun
http://dx.doi.org/10.5772/intechopen.95311
Authored by Helena Trindade Lopes and Ronaldo G. Gurgel Pereira

Contributors
Helena Trindade Lopes, Ronaldo G. Guilherme Gurgel Pereira

First published in London, United Kingdom, 2021 by IntechOpen
IntechOpen is the global imprint of INTECHOPEN LIMITED, registered in England and Wales, registration number: 11086078, 5 Princes Gate Court, London, SW7 2QJ, United Kingdom
Printed in Croatia

British Library Cataloguing-in-Publication Data
A catalogue record for this book is available from the British Library

Additional hard and PDF copies can be obtained from orders@intechopen.com

The Gynecological Papyrus Kahun
Authored by Helena Trindade Lopes and Ronaldo G. Gurgel Pereira
p. cm.
Print ISBN 978-1-83969-427-1
Online ISBN 978-1-83969-428-8
eBook (PDF) ISBN 978-1-83969-429-5

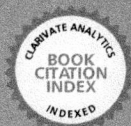

Meet the authors

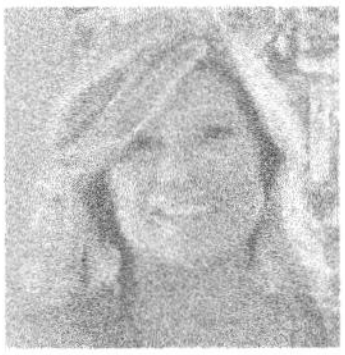

Maria Helena Trindade Lopes is Full Professor of Egyptology at the Faculty of Social Sciences and Humanities, Universidade Nova de Lisboa, Portugal, and Executive Coordinator of the Department of History. She is also the coordinator of the "Antiquity to its Reception" Group at CHAM - Humanities Center. She is the author of six scientific books, several chapters in collective works, two historical novels (*The Woman who Loved Pharaoh* and *Ramses II: The Living God who Conquered Lands and Hearts*), and a historical biography of Rome (*Rome, Eternal City*). She has also published more than 150 articles in journals and proceedings of scientific conferences. She was the director of the first Portuguese archaeological project in Egypt (Apriés Palace, in Memphis), which started in 2000 and ended in 2010.

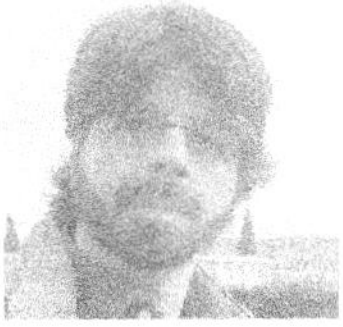

Ronaldo Guilherme Gurgel Pereira is a historian (Universidade Federal do Rio de Janeiro, Brazil) and archaeologist (Universidade Nova de Lisboa, Portugal). In 2010, he received a Ph.D. in Egyptology from the University of Basel, Switzerland. From 2012 to 2017, Dr. Pereira was a post-doctoral fellow at CHAM/FCSH – Universidade Nova de Lisboa. In 2018, he became an Onassis Fellow, hosted by the Department of Mediterranean Studies, University of the Aegean, Greece. In 2019, he became an auxiliary researcher at CHAM/FCSH – Universidade Nova de Lisboa. He teaches Middle Egyptian grammar, Hieratic, and disciplines regarding Egyptology, and the history of Phoenician and Greek expansion in the Mediterranean basin. In 2021, he was awarded a CAARI Scholar in Residence Fellowship.

Contents

Preface

Egyptology, as all sciences, is not closed in on itself, comfortably sealed off in ignorance of the world. It is true that for a long time she thought she was enjoying herself in splendid isolation, too imbued with being rewarded as an object of study with some of the most beautiful artistic and monumental achievements of humankind. But the narcissistic barriers with which she had surrounded herself inevitably gave way in the last third of the twentieth century. She could no longer remain insensitive to the great movements of ideas that agitated the world. Of these movements, one of the most important is certainly "feminism," understood in the broad sense as the realization that one half of humanity is unfairly assigned by the other to a secondary position. Feminism has resonated in Egyptology through personalities like Christiane Desroches Noblecourt, who promoted Pharaonic civilization in the world culture by crossing the Mediterranean to Tutankhamun to safeguard the temples of Nubia. It has also resonated through the proliferation of studies devoted to women in Pharaonic society. And it still resonates today, as evidenced by the initiative of Professor Maria Helena Trindade Lopes to propose a scientific edition of a treatise on gynecology that is a little less than four thousand years old. The medicine of Ancient Egypt was so famous that its practitioners were sometimes invited by some potentate of the Near East to help with cases considered hopeless. Even if only a small part of the Pharaonic medical literature has reached us, it is already substantial. The basic corpus was made available by the monumental series of works Grundriss der Medizin der Alten Ägypter under the aegis of the Berlin Academy. General and detailed studies on Egyptian medicine are also numerous, as many practitioners, suddenly transfixed by the vocation of Egyptologist, have striven to familiarize themselves with philology or even archaeology to contribute to the productions of professionals in this discipline.

What is more, in the luxuriance of the specialties participating in a rapidly developing archaeometry, paleo-medicines have particularly stood out with sometimes very spectacular results. Consider, among other things, the discovery of the assassination of Ramses III following a new examination of his mummy. Yet he had not been left behind after his discovery in the famous hiding place of Deir el-Bahri. As early as 1886, Gaston Maspero had undressed the mummy in the presence of the highest authorities. Then, other experts studied and even X-rayed it, without noticing the indisputable signs of a cut to the larynx 70-mm wide and extending to the bones of the fifth to the seventh vertebra, which must have caused immediate death. It was only detected ten years ago.

However, not all medical fields have benefitted from these great advances. Consider, for example, Egyptian gynecology. Fortunately, Professor Lopes was watching. Her perspicacity being sharpened by her feminist convictions, she soon realized the lack of notoriety from which this field suffered. To remedy this, she decided to present a scientific but very accessible edition of a major treatise on ailments specific to women from the Papyrus University College 32057, which is housed at the Petrie Museum of Egyptian Archeology, London. In this endeavor, she was joined by a young Brazilian Egyptologist, Ronaldo G. Gurgel Pereira. Both have worked together to publish the document in an almost ascetic ethic of rigour and sobriety, far from superfluous prolixity and self-promotional ranting in which sometimes some take pleasure. After describing the medium, the authors present the text in hieroglyphics, in transcription, and in translation. They also include a comment section that highlights cardinal data, classifies ingredients (medical materials), and evokes the mental processes at work. Finally, the authors include a valuable glossary that lists the lexical elements.

This little book elegantly contributes to the reconstruction of Pharaonic medicine and opens avenues to be explored. Beyond that, it is invested with a strong epistemological significance. Indeed, through him, in a country barely half a century previously confined under the bushel of an obscurantist dictatorship, the vigour of a young Egyptological school, turned towards the future, asserts itself. Its founder, Maria Helena Trindade Lopes, far from limiting herself to popularizing in her country a sort of epitome of our knowledge of Pharaonic Egypt, which was in itself a tour de force, wanted to contribute to the evolution of this same knowledge by opening it up to the great breadth of modernity. She was well-equipped to do this by her great historical and literary culture and by her constant sensitivity to a changing world. In the right spirit of the Carnation Revolution, she applied herself in Egyptology to taking off certain blinders.

Pascal Vernus
Directeur d'Études émérite,
École Pratique des Hautes Études,
IVe section,
Sorbonne

Dedication

"To Francisco, the love of my life.
To Luís Krus, my guardian angel.
I love you so much, always."

The Gynaecological Papyrus Kahun

Helena Trindade Lopes and Ronaldo G. Gurgel Pereira

Abstract

The Papyrus Kahun is oldest known Egyptian medical document addressing issues of midwifery, dating back to the second Millennium BC. Here it follows a study of the papyrus, featuring hieroglyphic text and its transliteration and translation versions. This work also features commentaries regarding the papyrus' medical substances and some linguistic evidences on the intimacy between spiritual and physical spheres in the Egyptian therapeutics. After the papyrus text, there is an Egyptian-English glossary.

Keywords: History of Medicine, Papyrology, Kahun, Ancient Egypt, Gynaecology

1. Introduction

The Gynaecological Papyrus Kahun[1], the oldest known medical papyrus, was discovered by W. M. Flinders Petrie in 1889, in a place near the modern city of Lahun, in Fayum [1][2]. The papyrus was in a very bad state of preservation, therefore it had to be carefully restored, in 1890, by Francis Griffith so he could, finally, be able to make the first hieroglyphic transcription of the hieratic text and its publication[3] still in 1898 [2]. Nowadays it is conserved in the Petrie Museum of Egyptian Archaeology, University College London (UC 32057), in London, United Kingdom.

The papyrus Kahun, dated from the kingdom of Amenemhat III, circa 1825 BCE[4] (Middle Kingdom, dynasty XII), is one of the biggest papyri of that period, with about 1 m long for 32 cm high, and features the oldest known treaty of gynaecology and obstetrics, which addresses issues such as fertility, pregnancy, contraception, and gynaecological diseases.

---

[1] The term Kahun was the name given by Petrie to the site of the city of Lahun, which, under the reign of Amenemhat III and his successors, would have been a very prosperous city.

[2] Nunn, 1996, p. 34.

[3] **The texts were published in facsimile, with hieroglyphic transcription and translation into English by Griffith**. CF. Griffith, F. Ll. (1898). *The Petrie Papyri: Hieratic Papyri from Kahun and Gurob*. London: Bernard Quaritch, p. 5–11 and pl. V-VI.

[4] A note on the reverse of the gynaecological papyrus is dated to the year 29 of Amenemhat III, *Ibidem*.

The work comprises three pages, is divided into 34 horizontal columns, oriented from the right to the left, that have a common format: begin with a brief report of the symptoms; then, the doctor is advised on how to approach the patient to present his diagnosis and, finally, treatment is suggested. However, no mention is made of the likely prognosis. This process of symptoms, diagnosis, report and treatment described makes up the various sections. Naturally, as in other medical works, Papyrus Kahun refers to an enchantment[5].

The suggested treatments are diverse and include fumigations, massages, and medications introduced into the body as pessaries or as a liquid to be drunk or rubbed on the skin. Donkey milk and perfumed oils are part of the medical material to be used in these procedures.

The text does not refer to any proposed surgery. The final paragraphs of the text are dedicated to pregnancy, presenting teachings related to conception which include the use of incense, fresh oil, dates, and beer, to contraception, suggesting the use of crocodile manure and also honey and natron and, again, gynaecological treatments.

After the publication of the Papyrus Kahun by Griffith [2] at the end of the XIX century, only in the second half of the XX century, the text is again the subject of study and publication within the scope of the most important investigation of medical papyri coordinated by H. Grapow [4], between 1954 and 1973. A hieroglyphic transcription of the papyrus Kahun is done in volume V and the translation and commentary of the text is presented in Volume IV.

In 1975, J. Stevens [5], presented an English translation of the text, and in 1995, Th. Bardinet, also presented his translation of the papyrus [6] and some comments on the text.

In 2002 Stephen Quirke published his transliteration and translation of the text online [7] and shared that translation again in the work he produces with M. Collier [8] in 2004.

Finally, in 2017, Didier Fournier introduced us to [9], where he performs the hieroglyphic transcription, transliteration, and translation of the papyrus as well as medical comments and lexical, syntactic and semantic considerations to the text. The work also reproduces the text in hieratic from facsimiles proposed by Griffith in 1898.

In addition to the publication and translation of the papyrus, the studies dedicated to the gynecological treatise presented in Papyrus Kahun are also very small. In 1952, C. D. Leake makes the first references in [10]. In 1992, C. Reeves in a small essay [11] also dedicates two pages to it. Four years later, J. F. Nunn in [1] introduces the papyrus and makes some comments on the text. Finally, in 2011, Lesley Smith published the latest article on the gynaecological papyrus Kahun [12]. Other references, in general works, although very reduced, happen in Strouhal, E., Vachala; B., Vymazalová [13], dated from 2014.

---

[5] In paragraph 30. The works on medicine in Ancient Egypt refer to the belief in a holistic dimension of life, in which the disease is understood, naturally, as a disturbance of an inner order that is reflected, a posteriori, physically [3]. Hence, the use of magical practices that could help harmonizes the patient.

DOI: http://dx.doi.org/10.5772/intechopen.98039

There are multiple semantic definitions and explanations for cure. Some of them are also based on mythical systems. In fact, this work assumes that cure is a double-folded concept. On one hand, the semantic meaning of cure manages to assert a cultural identity and a gender delimitation: Healthy vs. Diseased; Favoured by the gods vs. Abandoned by the gods, etc.

This approach of the Papyrus focuses on the so-called supernatural elements that, by any means are being mentioned in the therapeutics. We understand the separation between magic and medicine was unknown in Ancient Egypt, as they are the product of modern Egyptology problematization. The Egyptian medicine coordinates natural and supernatural elements in their therapeutics. Thus, we shall investigate the ontological specificities of the ancient Egyptian cure process. From the diagnosis to the therapeutics.

2. Commentaries

2.1 On the papyrus

The papyrus was composed in Hieratic, using a simple and direct language. It was probably compiled from some personal notes or a *vade mecum.*

There are 34 cases, along 3 columns of horizontal text, written from right to the left. Its first column (**Figure 1**) has 33.5 cm of height and starts the gynaecological tractate. This section has 29 short lines of text in good conditions.

The second column (**Figures 1** and **2**) has 38.5 cm of height and presents heavy damage on the central area of the page, between lines 26 and 59. So, only 7 lines out of its original 30 are complete. The second column also presents longer lines of text than the first one.

The third column (**Figure 2**) measures 33 cm of height and is also heavily damaged. Its 28 lines of text are the longest of the tractate. However, only one line is complete, from the beginning to the end. This column is divided into fragments A and B. Fragment B is just a small scrap with 4 incomplete illegible lines. Therefore, this work will deal with column 3 - fragment B only.

Another point of interest concerning column 3 is the transition to a totally different style of heading and organization of the treatments. That suggests column 1 and 2 have the same origin, while column 3 was copied from a different source.

For didactical matters, we decided to revert the text direction when we established the hieroglyphic matrix of this version. We also decided to present the

Figure 1.
Plate VI.1 (columns 1–2).

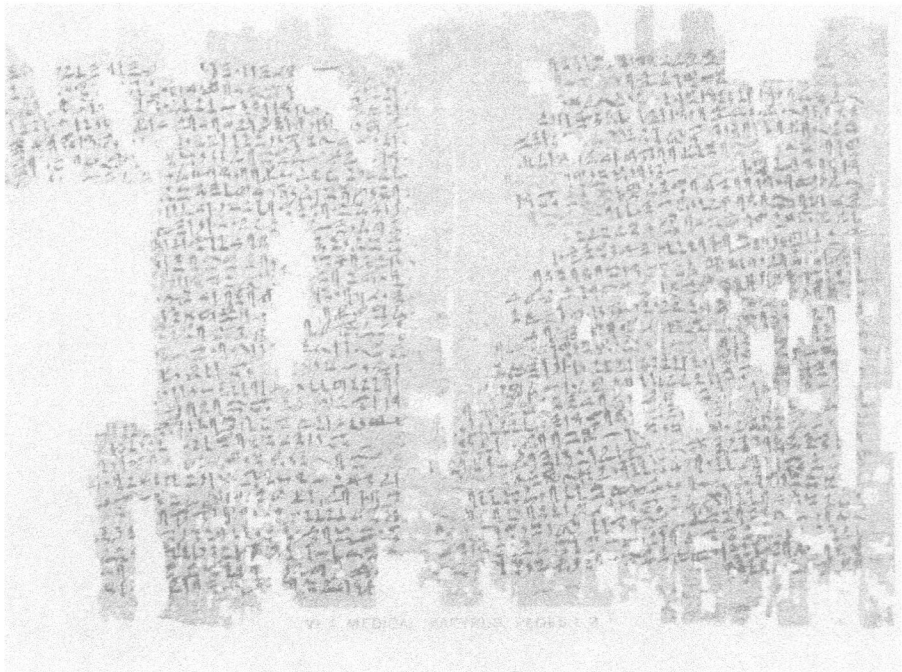

Figure 2.
Plate VI.2: (columns 2–3).

source in a format case-by-case for reasons of practicality. The present version of the text was originally built in Portuguese [14], and then, translated into English.

2.2 On the therapeutics

The 34 cases described in the papyrus are normally divided into mini-sections with the support of red ink. First, the disease is described. After making the diagnosis directly to the patient, a treatment is given.

The treatment presents the ingredients and, occasionally, the precise dosage of each element. Interestingly, this papyrus gives preference to generic measures, such as "spoon" or "jar". Then, the method of preparing the ingredients is concluded by the way the medicine must be applied to the patient.

Medicines are always taken orally, inserted into the vagina, or applied on the skin using massages or bandages. Fumigation seems to be the most common therapy, always incorporating various ointments with incense. There is great concern about therapy with the patient's uterus. Virtually all the diseases described are somehow linked to an origin in the uterus, and it is through the uterus that they seek to treat them [15].

The translation of this document took care to compare hieroglyphic versions established by British authors with Griffith's (1898) slides of hieratic text. It is interesting to note that all the translations previously cited reproduce the text in hieratic from facsimiles proposed by Griffith.

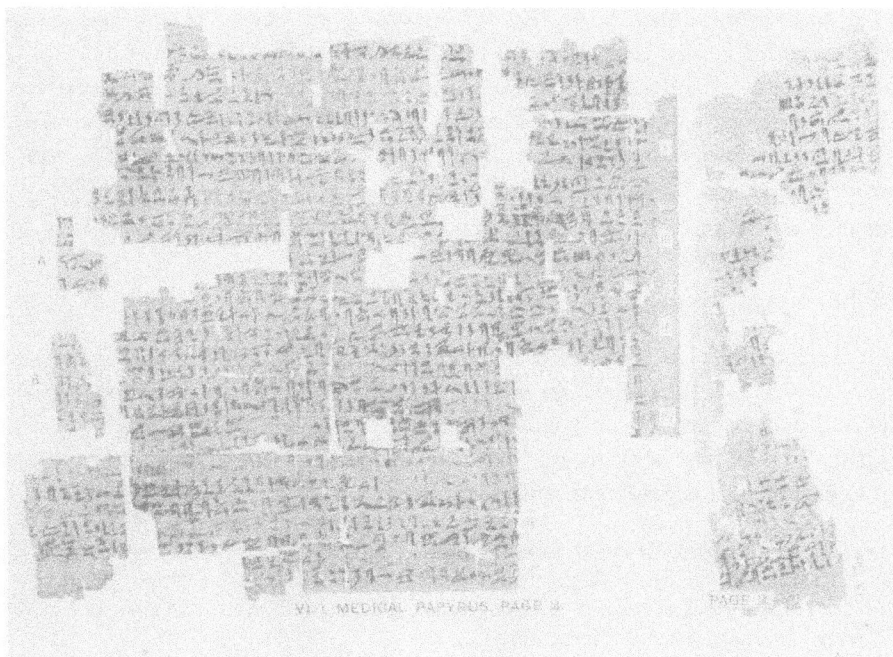

Hence, we found that the present version promoted "corrections" in the vocabulary proposed by previous works. The reader will find two diagnoses of incurable diseases (cases V and XIII), that are normally left aside by English translations. There is a short discussion on the spiritual dimension on Egyptian medicine (2.4). Further contributions are the identification of ingredients in the *materia prima* section (2.5), and of the procedure of verifying the patient's arterial pulse 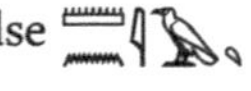 mnjꜣ (cases XXIX and XXXII).

2.3 P.Kahun as an educational text

From its 34 cases, there are 18 occurrences (1–17 & 25) where the papyrus actually can be used as a didactic textbook. In those texts, there is an approach aiming to guide the reader across each step of the therapeutic process. Such texts adopt the sequential sḏm.ḫr = f ("then, he should listen") providing the reader with the "what follow next" for each section. It is possible to summarize this pattern as the following:

- A heading to identify each new case (e.g. "A treatment for a woman who suffers A, B, C, etc."). A diagnostic is proposed to the reader. Then, the text concludes the first section with the recommendation: "then you should say to her" and announce the treatment.
- The diagnosis is described via a nominal identification sentence: "Disease-D" pw (this is a disease-D);
- Finally, the papyrus proceeds with the next step with the sayings: "then you must prepare for her" (here translated as "(then,) you should treat her), followed by the prescription of ingredients for each case and the right way of its application.

The didactic structure of this papyrus fits with the features of typology 4a, as proposed by [15], from which the table below is based on (**Table 1**).

I.	**Heading**	**šsꜣw s.t ḫr mn A, B, C etc.**	**"Treatment/Experiences on a woman who suffers from A, B, C, etc."**
II.	Investigation	*not present in typology 4a*	
III.	**Outcome**		
a	introduction	ḏd.ḫr = k r = s	"Then/consequently, you should say to her (on this regard)":
b = d	diagnosis = *causa*	"D" pw	"This is a D-disease!"
c	reasoning	*not present in typology 4a*	
IV.	**Treatment**	jrj.ḫr = k r = s	"Then/consequently, you should do for her (or even: 'then, you should do against it')".
Adaptation from Pommerening, 2014, p. 32.			

Table 1.
Text structure of typology 4a.

2.4 Regarding incurable diseases and spiritual influences

The Egyptian believed that both physical and the spiritual spheres of being were closely linked. The whole physical existence was understood as part of an eternal struggle between the cosmic forces of chaos and order. Simply put, a disease was nothing more than the physical manifestation of spiritual causes.

That said, a disease that was known to be intractable had its existence ascribed to some harmful spiritual force. These forces had several names, which traditionally Egyptologists translate as "demon", although that word does not have a direct equivalent in the Egyptian language.

In this papyrus we find only two therapies mentioning irreversible conditions. The term used to describe them is "bṯw" 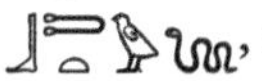, that is, a malefactor, according to lemma 10241 in [16]. The determinative 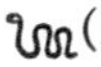(I 14) suggests a spiritual origin for that evildoer, meaning "demon".

That hieroglyph also is used as determinative of several minor spiritual powers [17], like – for instance - 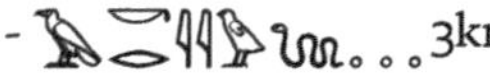 3kryw (chthonic gods or demons) in the Coffin Texts (II, 112e – Spell 105, S1C). However, it must be remarked the word bṯw is also synonymous with "incurable disease".

Due to a strong tendency to hide or diminish the importance of the spiritual in Egyptian medicine, the anglophone authors consulted translate btw as "worm" [7, 8] and "colic" [2], which is simply impossible, given the importance of the term at the conclusion of those cases.

Another connection between the physical and spiritual spheres in the Egyptian therapeutics is the usage of the verb 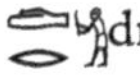dr. The word means equally "to expel" (case VIII: residuals from the body), "to drive away" (cases XXVIII and XXXIII: "pain") and is synonym with "to exorcize" (demons and disease demons) in the dictionary, lemna 39117 [16].

Generally speaking [3, 17, 18], a disease whose origin is ascribed to a spiritual origin sometimes can also/only be treated through magic formulas and prayers. Those incantations, or "heka" are normally dedicated to gods or minor spiritual entities, which would also be translated as "demons", but which are not necessarily evil forces. In this document, there is only a single case of enchantment, in the form of a prayer to Horus (case XXX), but the text is too damaged to let one understand exactly the possible usage of that magic formula.

2.5 On the medical *materia prima*[6]

The prescriptions of this papyrus normally combine ingredients of vegetal, animal and mineral origin in their different estates (solid, liquid, etc). Ingredients of mineral origin occur in less variety and those of animal origin are even rarer. There are multiple ways of preparation: fumigation, ingestion, etc.

[6] The term *materia medica* was first used by Dioscorides in *De Materia Medica* (1st century CE) and used ever since. However, since the Kahun papyrus predates Dioscorides, this work was encouraged to present another term for describing pharmaceutics, standing for the therapeutic features of any material used for treatment.

It is possible to divide the medical *materia prima* in two greater groups, by distinguishing ingredients of anthropic nature (it needs to be manipulated and transformed by man) *versus* ingredients that can be found in its natural milieu [18]. Thus, the Egyptian pharmacopeia is composed by hundreds of products collected and/or transformed from local flora and fauna.

In fact, Egyptian vegetal ingredients are mostly related to endemic specimens, However, out lack of knowledge about the Egyptian vegetal world posits a great obstacle to connect Egyptian names to actual plants. Therefore, traditional works by Egyptologists keep the Egyptian names untranslated [1, 18, 19].

A small lexicon follows, which complements the glossary at the end of this work.

Vegetal

- Vitex (*vitex agnus castus*). Case XIII - Its leaves, flowers, seeds and roots can be consumed with food or as an elixir. There is clinical evidence that it works to treat premenstrual tension [20].

- White Mullbery (*Morus alba*). Cases X, XII e XVI - Its extract has several medicinal properties. Here we highlight its effect with antibacterial, and in the treatment of hyperuricemia [21].

- Onion. Case XXVIII

- Beer. Case VI (to avoid it)

- Sweet beer. Cases XX e XXIV

- Fermented/ardent beer. Case X – Normally that term is translated as "djadjat-beer". It is a beer, fermented in some specific way. As the term djadjat is synonymous with "ardent", it can be a particularly strong beer.

- Cowpea (*Vigna unguiculata*). Case XXXIII

- Ripe figs. Case XVI

- Fruit (any). Cases III e XVII

- Fruit of the Onenu-tree. Case XX – Thus far an unidentified tree.

- Fruit of Egyptian balm (*Balanites aegyptiaca*). Case XVI - It was necessary to resort to the Hieratic text to propose the replacement of the unknown term 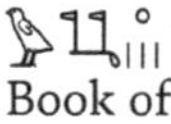 for 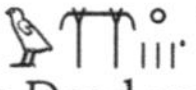. The sacred "ished" is a mythical tree referred to in the Book of the Dead spell 335. That passage mentions that it grows in the domain of the gods. A possible translation of "ished" is pistachio (*Pistacia vera*). However, the Egyptian balm is still used in Africa as a medicinal plant. It is employed to fight parasitic infection, headaches and liver disorders. Plus, its fruit is also indicated for stimulating lactation, while the bark of the tree is a natural abortive [22, 23].

- Fat/oil/unguent. Cases V e XVI

- Incense. Cases I, V, XX

- Watery porridge. Case VI
- Vegetal mucus of fermented mucilage. Case XIV
- Vegetal mucus of mixed mucilage. Case XIV
- Fermented vegetal mucus. Cases XX, XXI e XXIII
- Pulp of date (for syrups). Case XXIV
- Dregs of sweet beer. Cases XVII e XXVII
- Myrrh resin. Case XII
- Chufa (*Cyperus esculentus*). Cases III, X, XIII
- Oil/unguent (new). Cases I, IV e XX
- Grapes. Case XVI
- Date syrup. Cases XVII, XX e XXVII

Animal

- Cow milk. Cases III e XV
- Donkey/ass liver (fresh). Case I
- Honey. Case XXII
- Lard/fat of goose's leg. Case I
- Milk. Case XVIII

Mineral

- Donkey/ass urine. Case V
- Fermented beer. Case X
- Malachite powder. Case XV - This is a magical ingredient [18]. The mineral was used as a pigment for the green colour. In Egyptian, the same word can be used for naming "vigor", "vitality" and "freshness". Thus, by consuming the green pigment, one also acquired the properties that the magic pun (*rebus*) [24] provided in via "*sympatheia*".
- Mud. Case VII
- Natron. Case XXIII
- Spring water. Case XXV

Unidentified origin

- Emetic. Case XI (Its ingredients are not described)

- Fresh fat rancid oil. Case XII (It is not clear whether the fat is animal or vegetal).

2.6 Index of cases

COLUMN 1:

I – Pain in the eyes and throat; vision problems (lines 1–5);
II – Pain in the uterus (lines 5–8);
III – Pain in the lower limbs (lines 8–12);
IV – Abdominal and genital pain (lines 12–15);
V – Pain in the teeth and neck (lines 15–20);
VI – Pain in the limbs and eye sockets (lines 20–22);
VII – Pain in the feet and legs when walking (lines 23–25);
VIII – Pain in the throat, ears and groin; hearing problems (lines 25–27);
IX – Pain in the limbs, vulva and entire body (lines 27–29);

COLUMN 2:

X – Urinary problems (lines 30–34);
XI – A woman who cannot get out of her bed (lines 34–36);
XII – Pain in the legs (lines 36–40);
XIII – Pain in the legs and on the side of (a) ... (lines 40–47);
XIV – Thirsty for ... (lines 47–49);
XV – Swelling in the groin (lines 49–50);
XVI – Pain in the limbs and in the eye sockets (lines 51–54);
XVII – Hemorrhage ... (lines 54–59);

COLUMN 3:

XVIII – Sexual stimulant (line 1);
XIX – Pregnancy diagnosis (lines 2–3);
XX – Intoxication due to pregnancy medication (lines 3–6);
XXI – Prevention of ... (line 6);
XXII – Contraceptive (line 7);
XXIII – Treatment for ... (lines 7–8);
XXIV – Muscle cramp (trismus) of the uterus (lines 8–9);
XXV – Fever (lines 9–11);
XXVI – Pregnancy diagnosis (lines 12–14);
XXVII – Pregnancy diagnosis (lines 15–17);
XXVIII – Pregnancy diagnosis (lines 17–19);
XXIX – Pregnancy diagnosis (lines 19–20);
XXX – Pregnancy diagnosis (lines 20–23);
XXXI – Pregnancy diagnosis (lines 23–24);

DOI: http://dx.doi.org/10.5772/intechopen.98039

XXXII – Pregnancy diagnosis (lines 24–26);
XXXIII – Prevent trismus during childbirth (lines 25–26);
XXXIV – Urinary problem (lines 27–28).

3. Hieroglyphic text, transliteration and translation

COLUMN 1

No. I

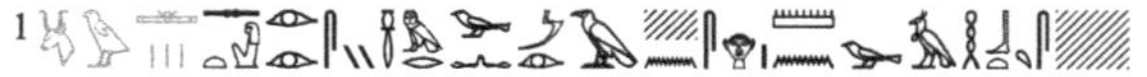

[1] šs3w s.t jr.tj=sj mr n(j) m33.n=s ḥr mn nḥb.t=s [...]

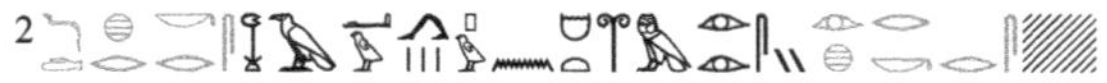

[2] ḏd.ḫr=k r=s ḫ3ʿw pw n jd.t m jr.tj=sj jr(j).ḫr=k r=s [...]

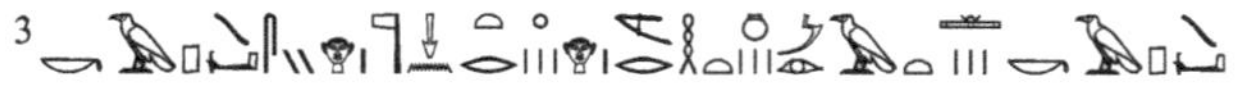

[3] k3p sj ḥr snṯr ḥr mrḥ.t-m3w.t k3p

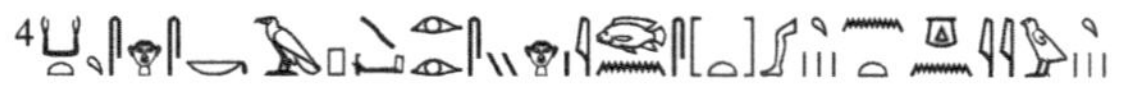

[4] k3.t=s ḥr=s k3p jr.tj=sj ḥr jns.wt n.t gnnw

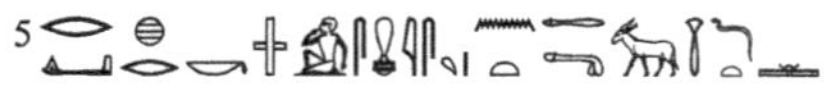

[5] rdj.ḫr=k wnm=s mjs.t n.t ʿ3 w3ḏ

Translation

[1] Treatment of a woman whose eyes are aching till she cannot see, on top of aches in her neck: [2] you should say to her: " it is discharges of the womb in your eyes!".

You should treat her: [3] fumigate her with incense and fresh oil, fumigating [4] her vulva with it, and fumigating her eyes with goose leg fat. [5] Then, you should give her to eat a fresh donkey liver.

No. II

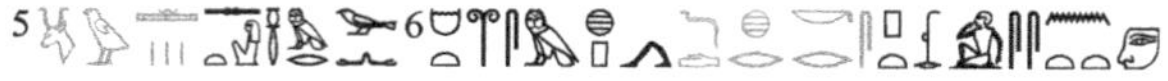

[5] šs3w s.t mr n(j) [6] jd.t=s m ḫp(j) ḏd.ḫr=k r=s ptr ssn.t(=ṯ)

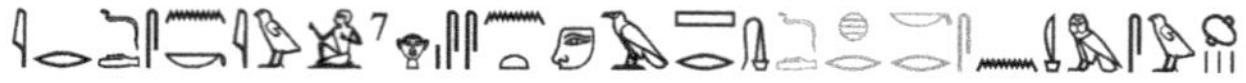

jr ḏd=s n=k jw=j [7] ḥr ssn.t 3šr ḏd.ḫr=k r=s nmsw

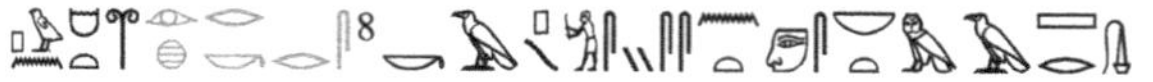

pw n jd.t jr(j).ḫr=k r=s [8] k3p sj ḥr ssn.t=s nb.t m 3šr

Translation

[5] Treatment of a woman in pain. Her [6] womb does not deliver (its period). You should say to her: "What do you smell?". If she says to you: "I [7] smell some roasting."

Then you should say to her: "This is some effusion of the womb!". You should treat her: [8] fumigate her with anything it smells like roast.

No. III

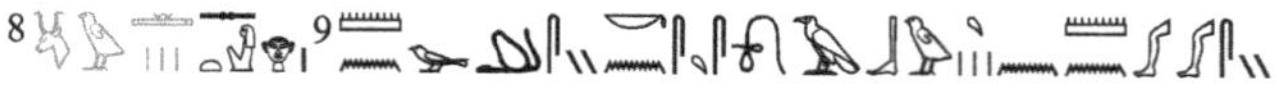

[8] šs3w s.t ḥr [9] mn pḥ(.wj)=sj kns=s w3bw n mn.tj=sj

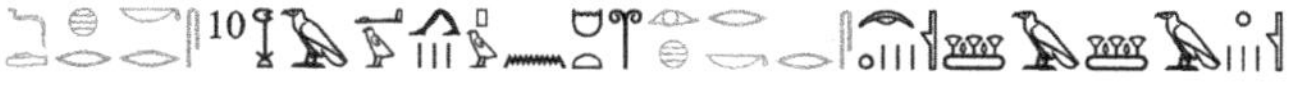

ḏd.ḫr=k r=s [10] ḫ3ʿw pw n jd.t jr(j).ḫr=k r=s wʿḥ š3š3 qd

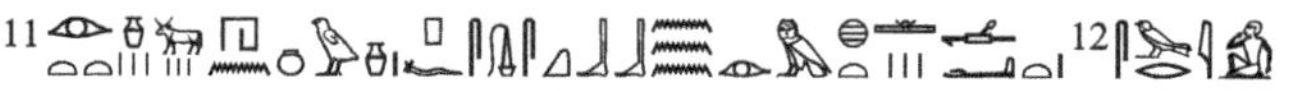

[11] jrṯ.t hnw 1 pf srf sqbb jr(j) m ḫtjw wʿ.t [12] swrj

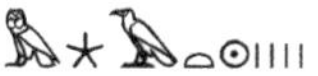

m dw3.t 4

Translation

[8] Treatment of a woman [9] aching in her hear, groin and perineum. You should say to her: [10] "These are discharges of the womb!".

Then, you should treat her: 1 qd of chufa (*cyperus esculentus*), 1 qd of fruit, 1 hin of [11] cow milk. Boil, let it cool down, [12] drink on 4 mornings.

No. IV

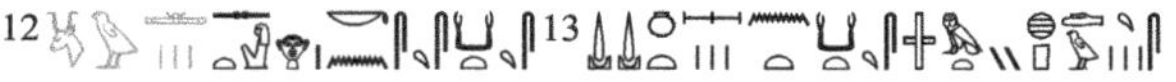

šs3w s.t ḥr kns=s k3.t=s [13] ḏ3ḏ3.t n.t k3.t=s jmj.tj ḫpd.w(j)=s(j)

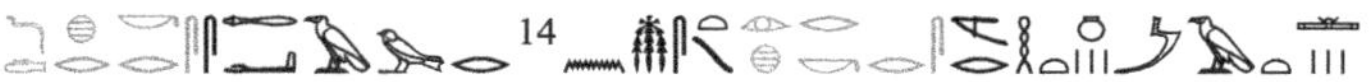

ḏd.ḫr=k r=s sʿ3 wr [14] n ms(j).t jr(j).ḫr=k r=s mrḥ.t m3w.t

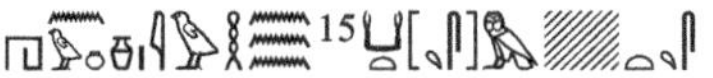

hnw 1 jwḥ [15] k3[.t=s] m [...].t=s

Translation

[12] Examination of a woman: regarding her groin, vulva and [13] the circuit of her vulva, between her buttocks. You should say to her: "Big dilatation [14] of birth!".

Then, you should treat her: 1 hin of fresh oil. Pour on her [15] vulva and her [...].

No. V

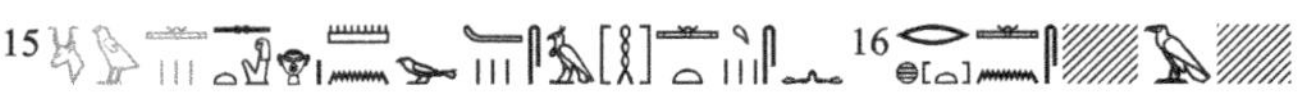

[15] šs3w s.t ḥr mn jbḥ.w=s nḥ.t=s n(j) [16] rḫ[.t] ns(q)

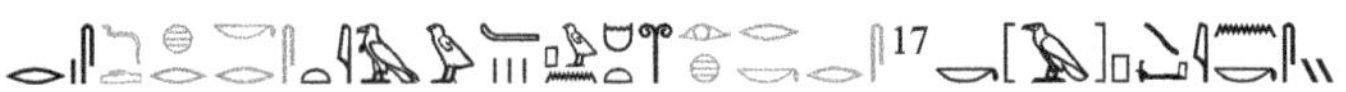

r(3)=s ḏd.ḫr=k r=s tj3w pw n jd.t jr(j).ḫr=k r=s [17] k[3]p.jn=k sj

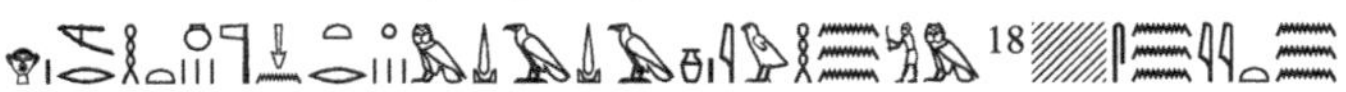

ḫr mrḥ.t snṯr m ḏ3ḏ3w jwḥ m [18] [...]=s mwy.t

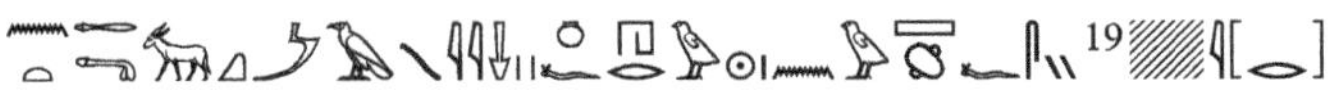

n.t ʿ3 qm3y snw=f hrw 1 n wš=f sj [19] [...] j[r]

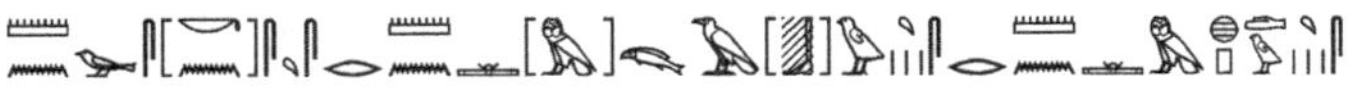

mn=s [kn]s=s r mn [m] ḫ3[b]w=s r mn m ḫpd.w=s

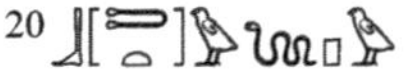

[20] bṯw pw

Translation

[15] Treatment of a woman aching in her teeth and throat to the point that she [16] cannot bite or [...] her mouth. You should say to her: "It is a trismus of the womb!".

Then, you should treat her [17]: after fumigating her with incense in a djadjaw-pot, pour on her [18] [...] the urine of a donkey that has "created its second" the day after it was feed. [19] If her pain is situated from the bellybutton to her buttocks, it is a demon (untreatable).

No. VI

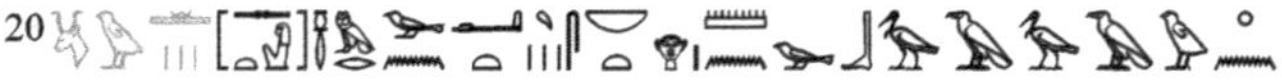

[20] šs3w [s.t] mr n ꜥ.wt=s nb.t ḥr mn b3b3w n

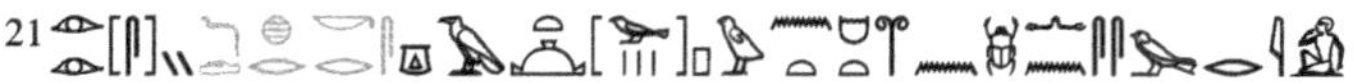

[21] jr.tj=sj ḏd.ḫr=k r=s g3.t pw n.t jd.t n ḫpr nn sswrj

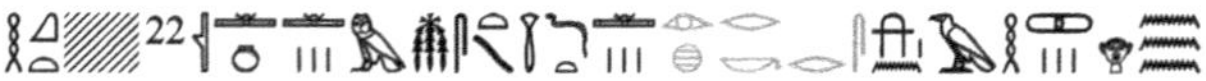

ḥnq.t [...] [22] qd m ms(j).t w3ḏ.t jr(j).ḫr=k r=s ḥsb 1 n 3ḥ ḥr mw

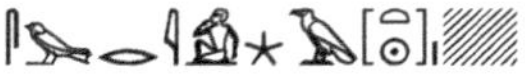

swrj dw3[.t] 1 [+ x]

Translation

[20] Treatment of a woman aching her limbs and [21] eye-sockets. You should say to her: "It is some deprivation of the womb! No beer-drinking [22] shall grant a healthy birth!".

Then, you should treat her: 1 hsb of watery porridge. Drink it on 1 [+ x] mornings.

No. VII

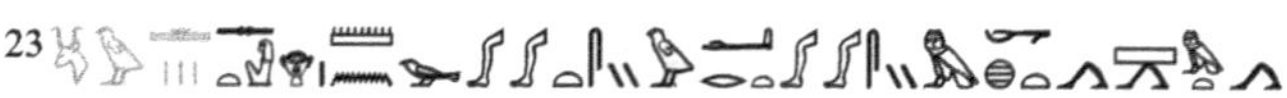

[23] šs3w s.t ḥr mn rd.wj<t>=sj wꜥr.tj=sj m-ḫ.t šm.t

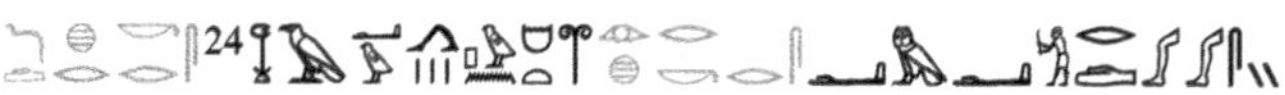

ḏd.ḫr=k r=s [24] ḫ3ꜥw pw n jd.t jr(j).ḫr=k r=s ꜥmꜥm rd.wj=sj

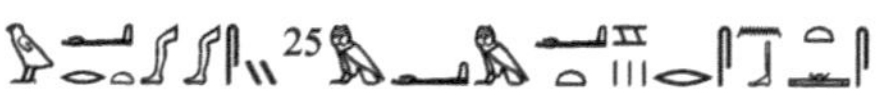

wꜥr.tj=sj [25] m ꜥmꜥ.t r snb.t=s

Translation

[23] Treatment of a woman aching in her feet and legs after a walk. You should say to her: "It is a [24] discharge of the womb!".

Then, you should treat her: rub her feet and legs [25] with mud until she is well.

No. VIII

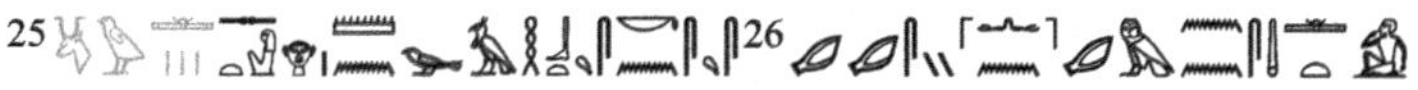

šs3w s.t ḥr mn nḫb.t=s kns=s [26] msḏr.wj=sj (n)n sḏm.n=s mdw.t

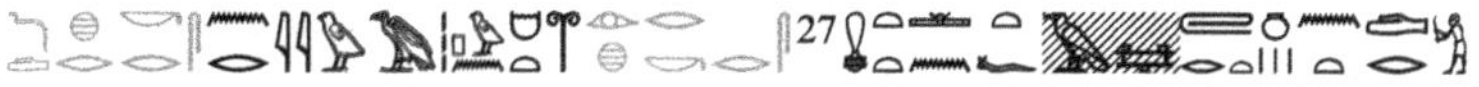

ḏd.ḫr=k r=s nrw pw n jd.t jr(j).ḫr=k r=s [27] mjtt n tf3 pḫr.t n.t dr

sḥ3w n jd.t [...]

Translation

[25] Treatment of a woman aching her throat, groin and (so much) [26] her ears that she does not hear what it is said. You should say to her: “This is a tremor of the womb!”.

Then, you should treat her with [27] the same prescription for expelling residuals from the womb [...].

No. IX

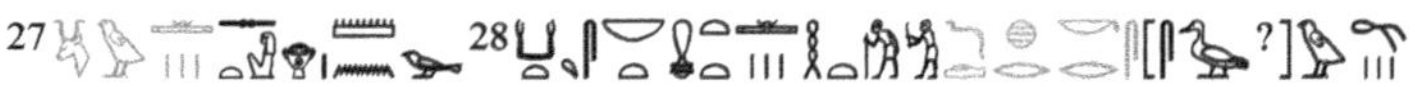

[27] šs3w s.t ḥr mn [28] k3.t=s nb.t mjtt ḥw(j).t ḏd.ḫr=k r=s [...]

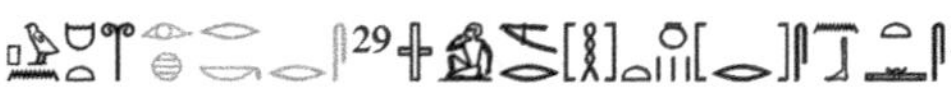 End of Column 1

pw n jd.t jr(j).ḫr=k r=s [29] wnm mr[ḥ].t=s [r] snb.t=s

Translation

[27] Treatment of a woman aching in her [28] vulva and all her limbs, as if she had been beaten. Then, you should say to her: “It is [...] of the womb”.

Then, you should treat her: [29] eating fat (a fat diet) until she is well.

COLUMN 2

No. X

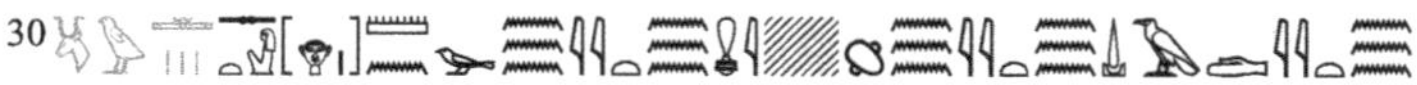

30 šsꜣw s.t [ḥr] mn mwy.t mj [...] mwy.t ḏꜣdy.t

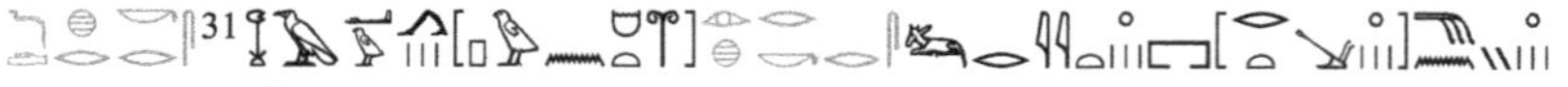

ḏd.ḫr=k r=s 31 ḫꜣw [pw n jd.t] jr(j).ḫr=k r=s jwry.t pr[.t]-šnj

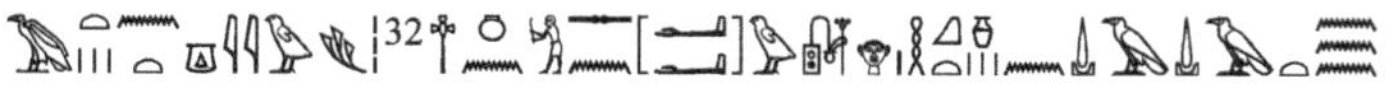

mw.t n.t gyw 32 nḏ sn[ꜥꜥ]w ḥr ḥnq.t n ḏꜣḏꜣ.t

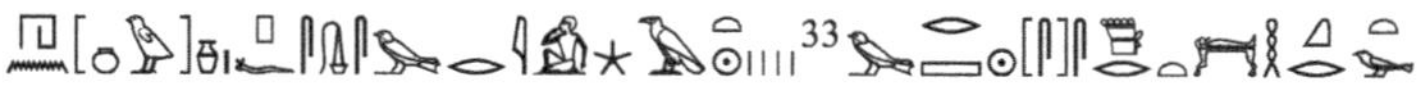

hn[w] 1 ps swrj dwꜣ.t 4 33 wrš[=s] sḏr.t ḥqr.t

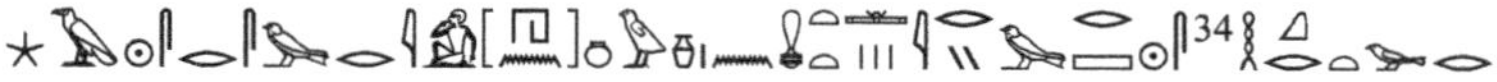

dwꜣ(.t)=s r swrj [hn]w 1 n-mjtt jrj wrš=s 34 ḥqr.t r

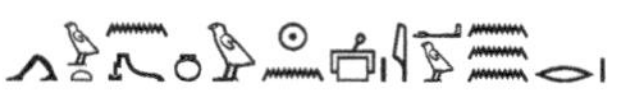

jw(j).t nw sꜣ - jꜥw-r(ꜣ)

Translation

30 Treatment of a woman aching when urinating, as if [...] burning/fermented. You should say to her: "This is 31 discharges of the womb!".

Then, you should treat her: beans of white mulberry (*morus alba*) and chufa (*cyperus esculentus*). 32 Grind it and dilute in 1 hin of fermented beer. Boil and drink on 4 mornings. May she 33 spend the day fasting on her bed after drinking 1 hin of the same. May she spend the day 35 fasting until the moment of washing her mouth.

No. XI

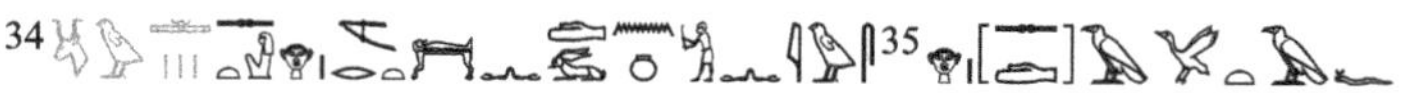

34 šsꜣw s.t ḥr mr.t n(j) dwn=s n(j) jw=s 35 ḥr [sd]ꜣ.t=f

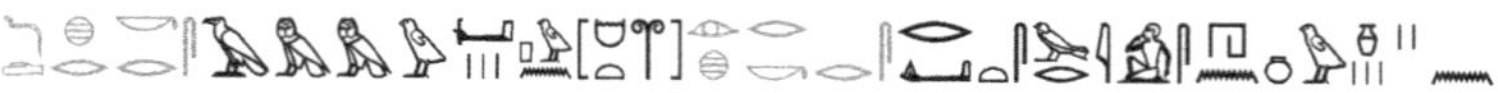

ḏd.ḫr=k r=s ꜣmmw pw n [jd.t] jr(j).ḫr=k r=s rdj.t swrj=s hnw 2 n

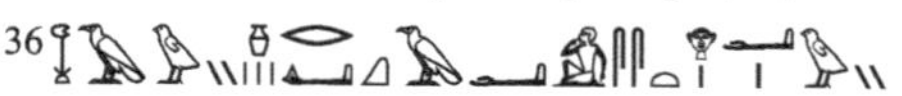

36 ḫꜣwj rdj qꜣꜥ=s st ḥr-ꜥ.wj

Translation

34 Treatment of a woman bed-bound, without standing or 35 moving. You should say to her: "This is a weakness of the womb!".

Then, you should treat her: let her drink 2 hin of 36 emetic and have her to throw it up at once!

No. XII

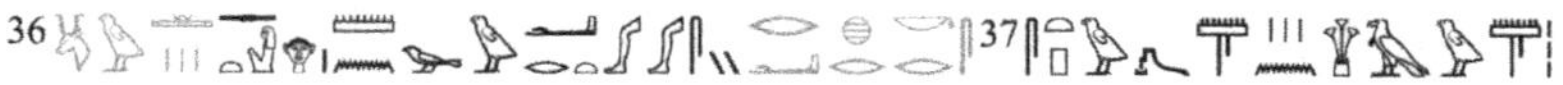

[36] šs3w s.t ḫr mn wꜥr,tj=sj rdj.ḫr=k r=s [37] stpw n ḥ3tjw

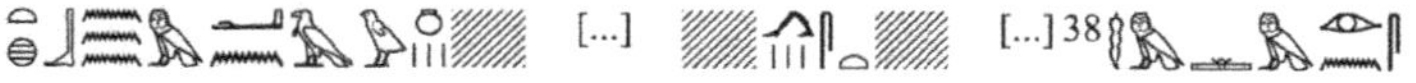

tḫb m ꜥntjw [...] st [...] [38] nḏm m jr(j).n=s

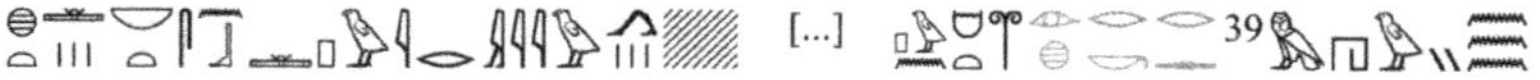

ḫ.t nb.t snb pw jr jjjw [...] pw n jd.t jr(j).ḫr=k r=s [39] mhwj

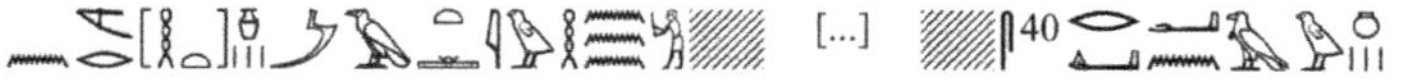

n mr[ḥ.t] m3.t jwḥ [...]=s [40] rdj ꜥntjw

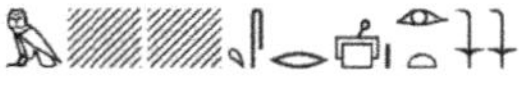

m [...]=s r-s3 jrj.t nn

Translation

[36] Treatment of a woman aching in her legs. You should give to her [37] bandages soaked in resin of myrrh [...] it [...]. [If ...] [38] sweet, after she has done all that, it means health. If what leaves is [...] "This is [...] of the womb!".

Then, you should treat her: [39] fresh rancid oil. Pour over her [...]. Place resin of myrrh on her [...] after doing this.

No. XIII

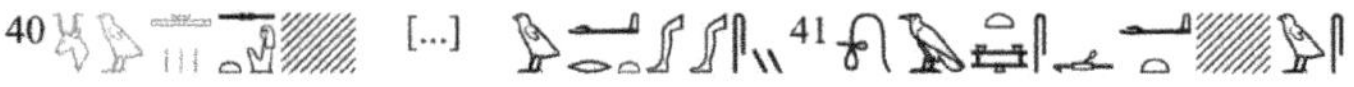

[40] šs3w s.t [...] wꜥr.tj=sj [41] w3.t=s wꜥ.t [...]w=s

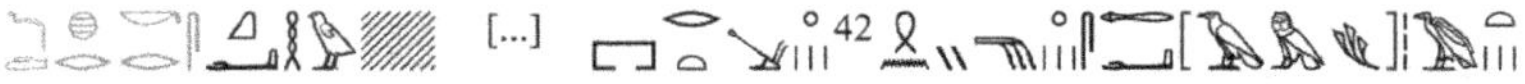

ḏd.ḫr=k r=s qꜥḥw [...] pr.t- [42] šnj sꜥ3m mw.t

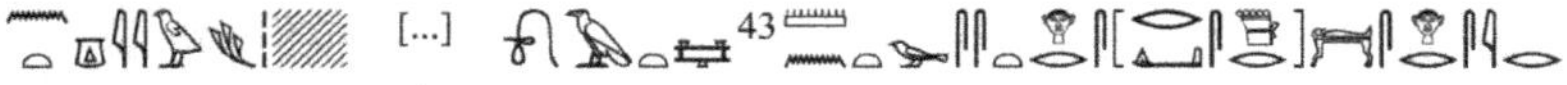

n.t gyw [...] w3.t [43] mn.t=s st ḥr=s [rdj sdr]=s ḥr=s jr

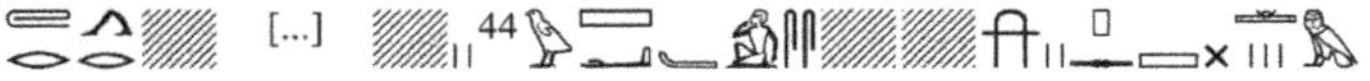

pḫr r [...] 2 [44] wšꜥ=s s[...] ḥsb 2 psš m

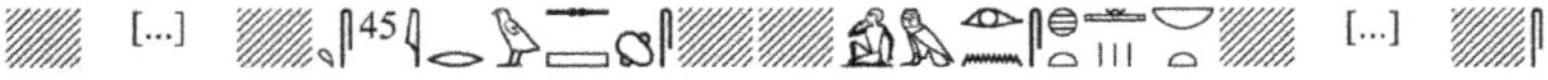

[...]=s [45] jr wš=s [...] m jr(j).n=s ḫ.t nb.t [...]=s

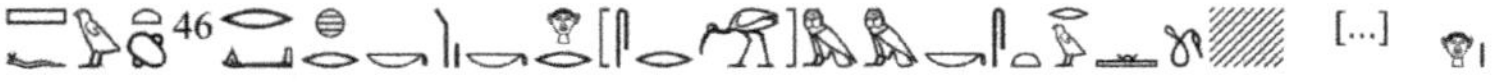

šfw.t [46] rdj.ḫr=k ḏb3=k ḥr=[s r gm]m=k st rwḏ(.t) [...] ḥr

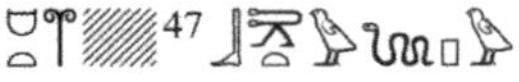

jd.t [...] [47] bṯw pw

Translation

[40] Treatment of a woman [...] her legs and on [41] one side of her [...]. You should say to her: "(This is a) bulge [...]".

[Then you should treat her:] beans of white [42] mulberry (*morus alba*), chaste-tree (*vitex agnus castus*), and chufa (*cyperus esculentus*) [...] on the side she [43] aches, and let her lay down on her side. If [...] circulates [...] 2, [44] divided in her [...]. [45] If she itches [...] it means she did all things [...] a swollen, [46] then you should place your finger on it until you find it firm [...] on the womb, it is a demon (untreatable).

No. XIV

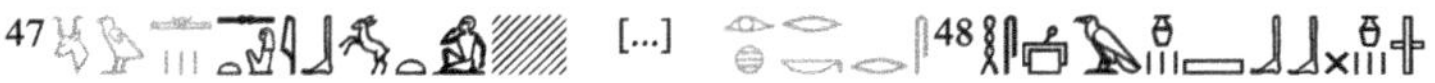

[47] šsꜣw s.t jb.t [...] jr(j).ḫr=k r=s [48] ḥsꜣ šbb jmj

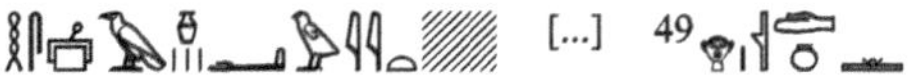

ḥsꜣ ꜥwy.t [...] [49] ḫr-qd

Translation

[47] Treatment of a woman thirsting [...].

Then, you should treat her: [48] vegetal mucus of a mixed mucilage and vegetal mucus of a fermented mucilage [...] [49] completely.

No. XV

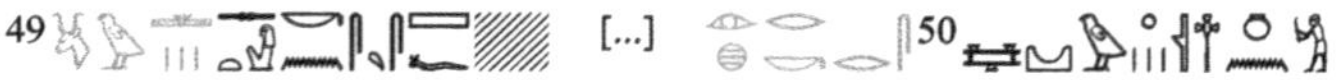

[49] šsꜣw s.t kns=s šf(w) [...] jr(j).ḫr=k r=s [50] wꜣḏw qd (1) nḏ

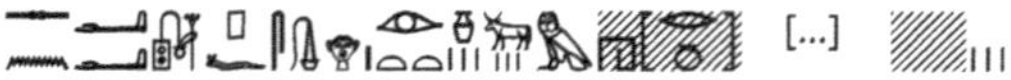

snꜥꜥ ps ḥr jrt.t mh[r] [...] 3 (+ x)

Translation

[49] Treatment of a woman with a swollen groin [...].

Then, you should treat her: [50] (1) qd of malachite powder. Grind, refine and boil in 1 jar of cow milk [...] 3 [+ x].

No. XVI

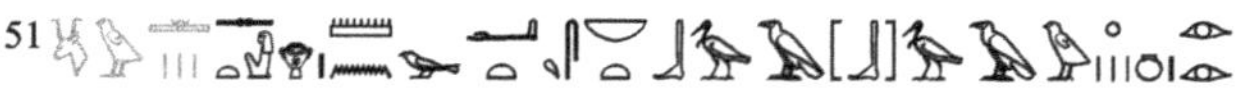

[51] šsꜣw s.t ḥr mn ꜥ.t nb.t bꜣbꜣw.w nw jr.tj

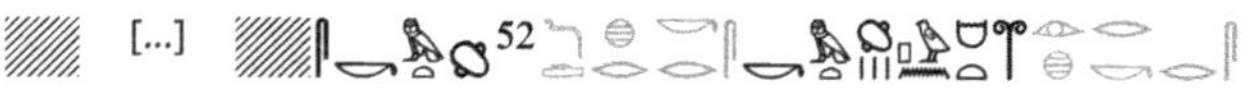

[...]=s km.t [52] ḏd.ḫr=k r=s km.wt pw n jd.t jr(j).ḫr=k r=s

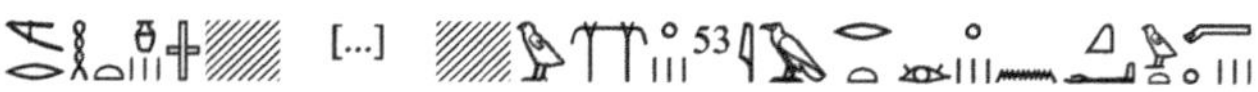

mrḥ.t jmj [...] jšd [53] jꜣr.t nqꜥ.wt

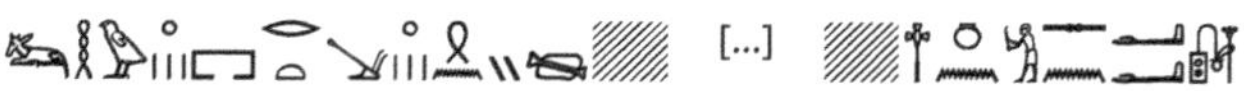

jwḥw pr.t-šnj […] nḏ sn[cc]

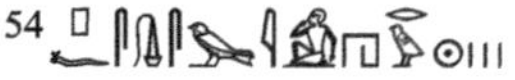

[54] ps swrj hrw 3

Translation

[51] Treatment of a woman aching all her limbs and eye-sockets […] her a disease. Then you should say to her: “This is a disease of the womb!”.

[52] Then, you should treat her: oil, fruit of Egyptian balm (*balanites aegyptiaca*), [53] grapes, ripe figs and beans of white mulberry (*morus alba*) […]. Grind, refine and [54] boil. Drink for 3 days.

No. XVII

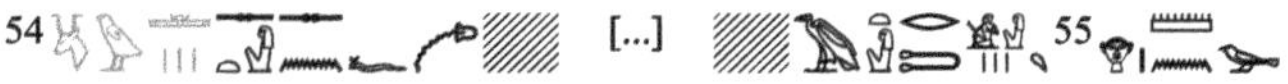

[54] šs3w s.t snf […] mw.t-rmṯ [55] ḥr mn

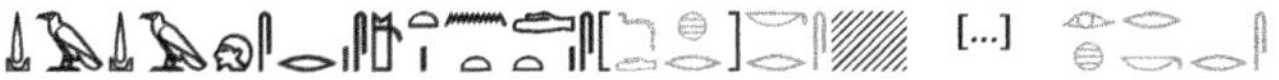

ḏ3ḏ3=s r(3)=s ḥn.t n.t d.t=s [ḏd.ḫr]=k r=s […] jr(j).ḫr=k r=s

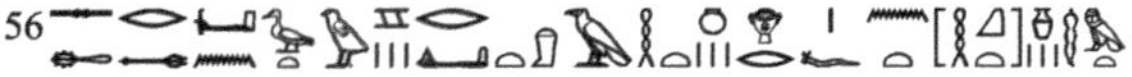

[56] sḫr n=s s3ṯw rdj t3ḥ.t ḥr=f n.t [ḥnq.t]-nḏm.t

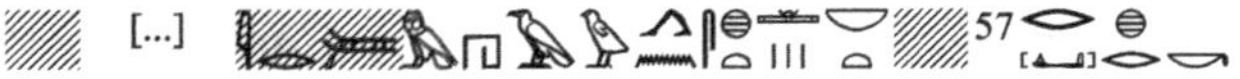

[…] jr tm h3w.n=s ḫ.t nb.t […] [57] r[dj].ḫr=k

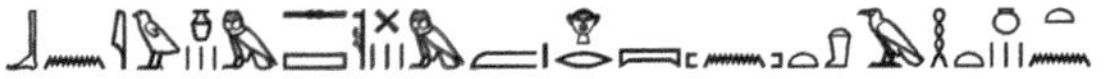

bnjw m sš m-gs-ḥr(j) [n] t3ḥ.t tn

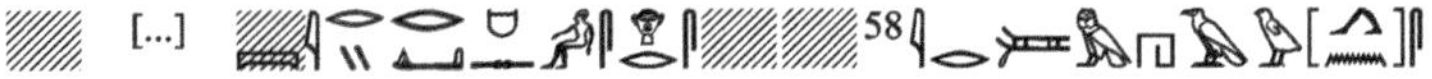

[…] (ḥrj) jrj rdj ḥms=s ḥr=s […] [58] jr tm h3w [n]=s

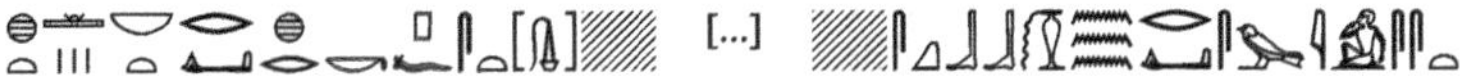

ḫ.t nb.t rdj.ḫr=k ps.t […] sqbb rdj swrj=s st

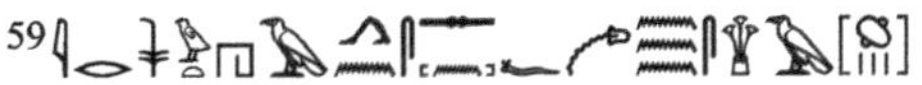

[59] jr swt h3 n=s s[n]f=s sḥ3w

 [...] End

r(3)-pw […]

Translation

[54] Treatment of a woman bleeding […] mother of persons, [55] aching in her head, mouth and wrists. You should say to her: […].

Then, you should treat her: [56] prepare for her a spot on the ground and place on it the dregs of sweet beer. […]. If nothing leak out from her, [57] you should place date syrup over the top of that as a nest […]. Let her seat on it […]. [58] If nothing leak out from her, you should cook […] let it cool. Make her drink it. [59] If, however, blood or residuals leak from her, [… .].

COLUMN 3

No. XVIII

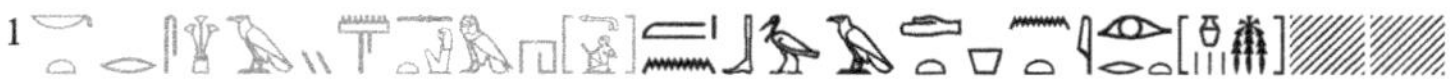

[1] k.t r sḥꜣj s.t m hꜣj gs n bꜣd.t n.t jrt.t [ms ...]

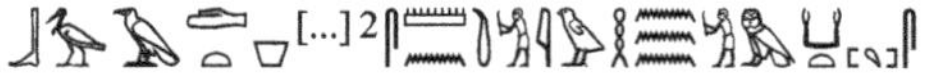

bꜣd.t [...] [2] smn jwḥ m kꜣ.t=s

Translation

[1] Another one, for unveiling a woman while copulating. Half of a scoop of milk [...] scoop [...] [2] let it stabilize. Pour it in her womb.

No. XIX

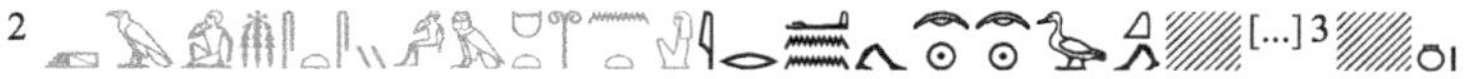

[2] sjꜣ ms.tj=sj m jd.t n.t s.t jr ʿnn ꜣbd ʿq [...] [3] [...] nw

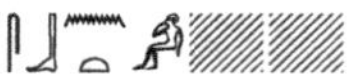

sbn.t [...]

Translation

[2] Noticing a child inside the womb of a woman. If month ends and month starts [...] of nursing [...] [3] [...].

No. XX

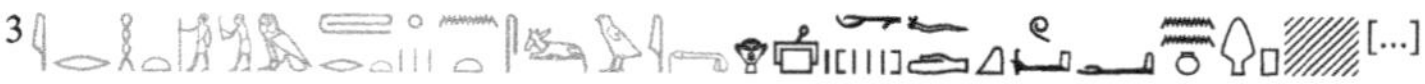

[3] jr ḥw(j).t m pḫr.t n.t sjwj ḫr-sꜣ fdq ʿnnw.t [p ...]

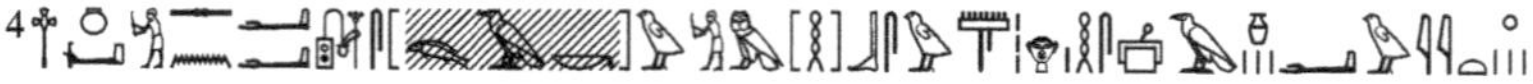

[4] nḏ snʿʿ s[ḫꜣk]w m [ḥ]bsw ḥr ḥsꜣ-ʿwy.t

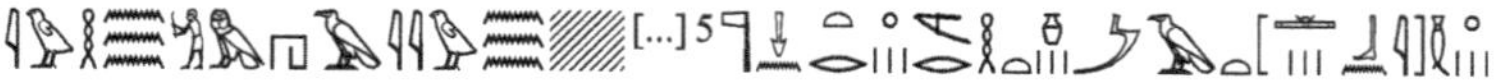

jwḥ m hꜣyw [...] [5] snṯr mrḥ.t [bnj]w

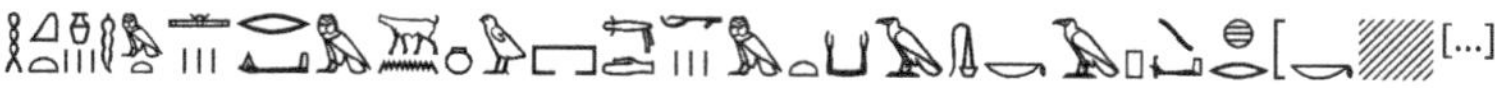

ḥnq.t nḏm.t rdj m-ḫnw šdj m tkꜣw kꜣp.ḫr[=k ...]

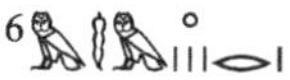

[6] m nḏm-r(ꜣ)

Translation

[3] If a woman was stricken by some prescription for pregnancy. After severing the fruit of an Onnw-tree, [...] [4] Grind and refine, by filtering with a clothing with fermented vegetal mucus. Bath with waves [...]. [5] Incense, new oil, date syrup and sweet beer. Give it to a burning vessel. Then, you should burn [...] [6] as a sweetener of the mouth.

No. XXI

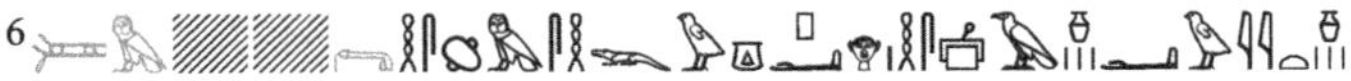

6 tm […] ḥs msḥ wgp ḥr ḥs3 ʿwy.t

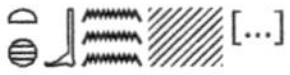

tẖb […]

Translation

6 For preventing […]. Crocodile dung. Pound it with fermented vegetal mucus, immersed (in) […].

No. XXII

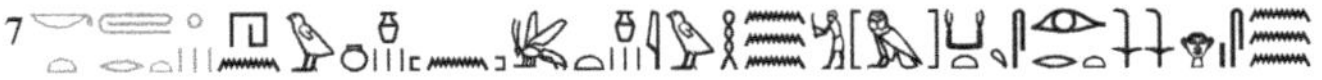

7 k.t pẖr.t hnw [n] bj.t jwḥ [m] k3.t=s jr(j).t nn ḥr sḥm

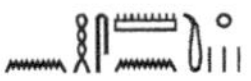

n ḥsmn

Translation

7 Another prescription: (1) hin of honey. Pour it into her vulva. This is to be done together with a natron contraceptive.

No. XXIII

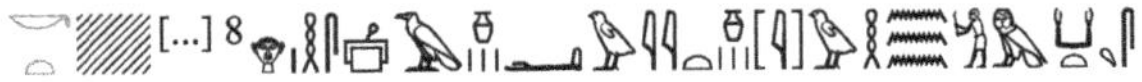

k.t […] 8 ḥr ḥs3 ʿwy.t [j]wḥ m k3.t=s

Translation

Another one […]. 8 with fermented vegetal mucus. Sprinkle inside her vulva.

No. XXIV

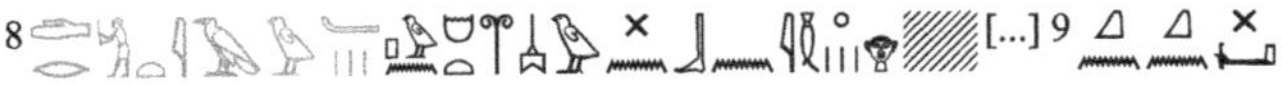

8 dr tj3w pw n jd.t wḏʿ n bnjw ḥr […] 9 qnqn

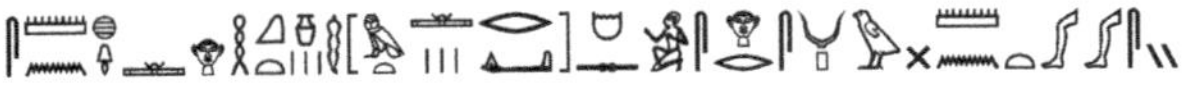

smnḫ ḥr (sic) ḥnq.t nḏm.t rdj ḥms(j)=s ḥr=s wpw mn.t(j)=sj

Translation

8 This is for removing muscular pains of the womb. Date palm pulp with […]. 9 Crush it and reduce it in sweet beer. Let her sit on it with her legs apart.

No. XXV

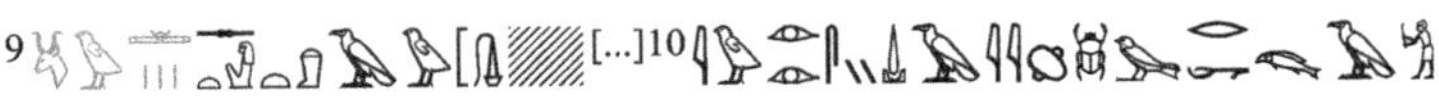

9 šs3w s.t t3w […] 10 jw jr.tj=sj ḏ3y(.t) ḫpr-wr ẖ3

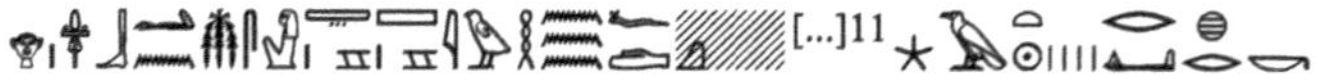

ḥr jꜣb n ms(j)-tꜣ š jwḥ fdq [...] [11] dwꜣ.t 4 rdj.ḫr=k

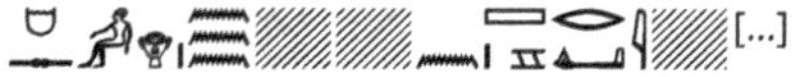

ḥms=s ḥr mw n š rdj [j ...]

Translation

[9] Treatment of a woman burning (with fever) [...], [10] her eyes are harmed. Wild carrot. Spread on the left side of the "msta" (birth brick?) with spring water. Sprinkle and sever [...]. [11] 4 mornings. Then, you should let her siting on the water of [...] spring water. Give [...].

No. XXVI

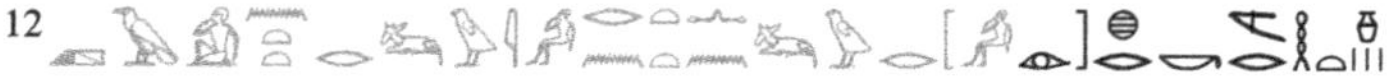

[12] sjꜣ ntt r jwj r ntt nn jwr [jr(j)].ḫr=k mrḥ.t

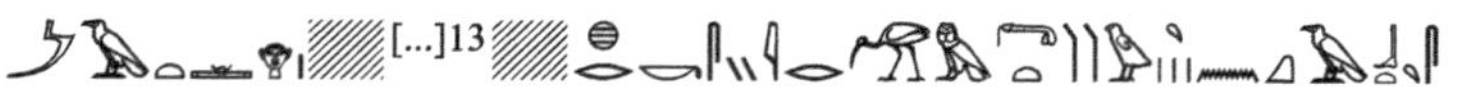

mꜣ.t ḥr [...] [13] [...].ḫr=k sj jr gm(j) mtjw n qꜣb.t=s

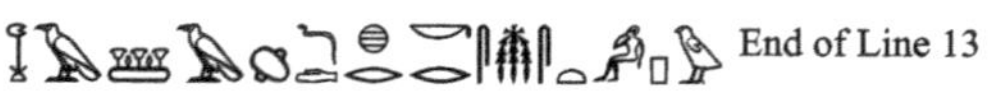

ḫꜣšꜣ ḏd.ḫr=k r=s ms(j).t pw

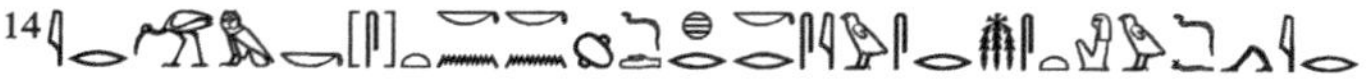

[14] jr gm(j)=k [s]t knkn ḏd.ḫr=k r=s jw=s r ms(j).t wḏf jr

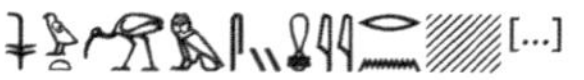

swt gm(j) sj mj jrn[...]

Translation

[12] Determining a woman who shall conceive from one who shall not. You should prepare: new fat and [...]. [13] Then, you should [...]. If the muscles of her breasts are showing some bulging, you should say to her: "This is pregnancy!". [14] If you find it in a normal state, you should say that she will give birth late. However, if you find her something like [...].

No. XXVII

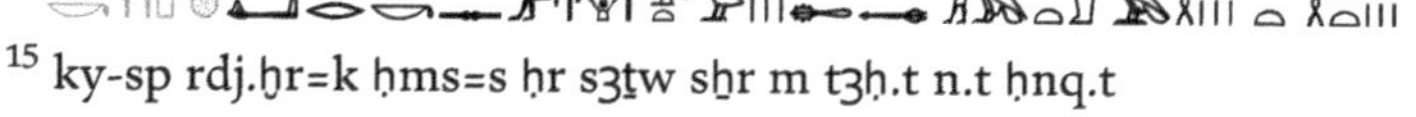

[15] ky-sp rdj.ḫr=k ḥms=s ḥr sꜣṯw sḫr m tꜣḥ.t n.t ḥnq.t

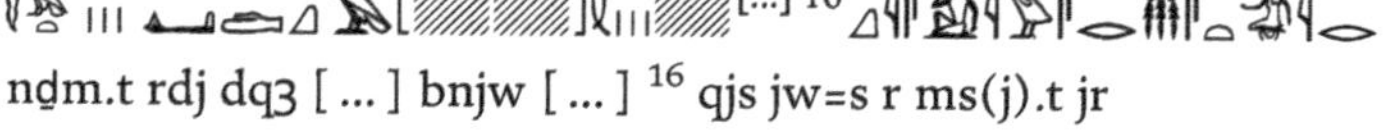

nḏm.t rdj dqꜣ [...] bnjw [...] [16] qjs jw=s r ms(j).t jr

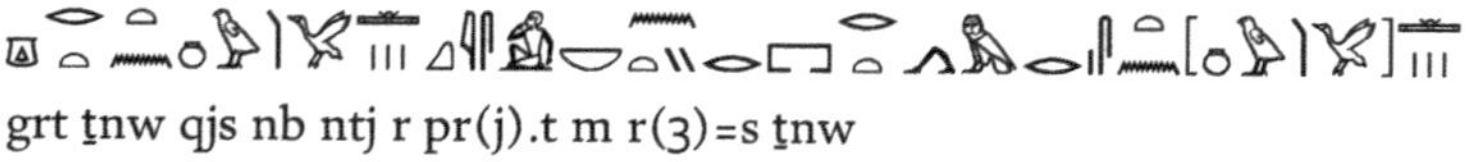

grt ṯnw qjs nb ntj r pr(j).t m r(ꜣ)=s ṯnw

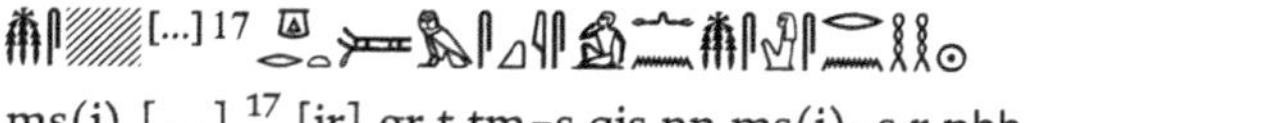

ms(j) [...] [17] [jr] gr.t tm=s qjs nn ms(j)=s r nḥḥ

Translation

[15] Another time. You should let her siting on the ground prepared with dregs of sweet beer. Put some fruit [...] date syrup [...]. [16] vomits, she will give birth. Indeed, every time some vomit leaves her mouth it means a birth. [17] However, if there is no vomit at all she will never give birth.

No. XXVIII

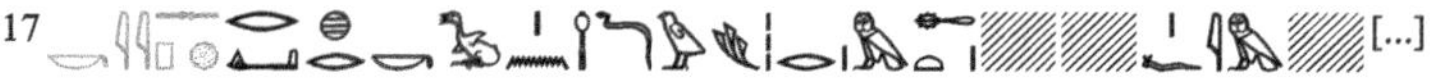

[17] ky-sp rdj.ḫr=k ṯ3 n ḥḏw r(3) m ḫ.t [...]=f jm [...]

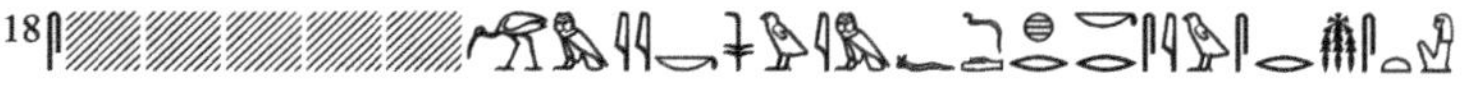

[18] s[...] gmy=k sw jm=f ḏd.ḫr=k r=s jw=s r ms(j).t

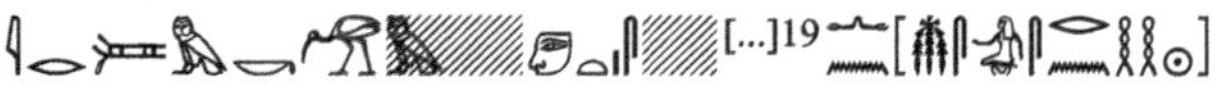

jr tm=k gm(y=k) [...] ḫn.t=s [...][19] nn [ms(j)=s r nḥḥ]

Translation

[17] Another time. You should give an onion bulb on the mouth (entrance) of her belly [...] it [...] there. [18] [...]. (If) you find in it, then you should say to her that she will give birth. If you do not find [...] her face [...] [19] she will never give birth.

No. XXIX

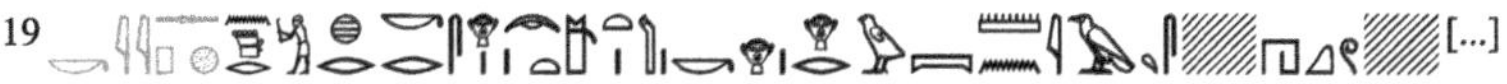

[19] ky-sp nḏr.ḫr=k r=s ḥr šsp=s ḥn.t-dbꜥ=k ḥr-ḥrjw mnj3=s [...] (n)hq [...]

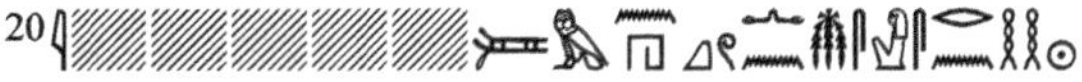

[20] j[r ...] tm nhq nn ms(j)=s r nḥḥ

Translation

[19] Another time. You should press her hand with the tip of your finger on her point of pressure. [...]. Pain [...]. [20] If [...] there is no pain, she will never give birth.

No. XXX

[20] ky-sp bḥs pwy n Ḥr [...] [21] [...] jw=j ḥr [...] Ḥr ṯs-pḫr(w)

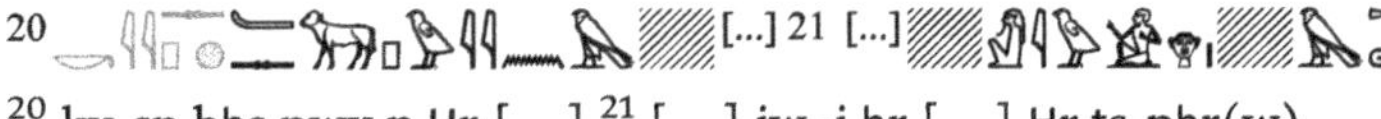

h3(j)=k r bw n [...]=k jm ḏd.tw r(3) [...] [22] [...] jr

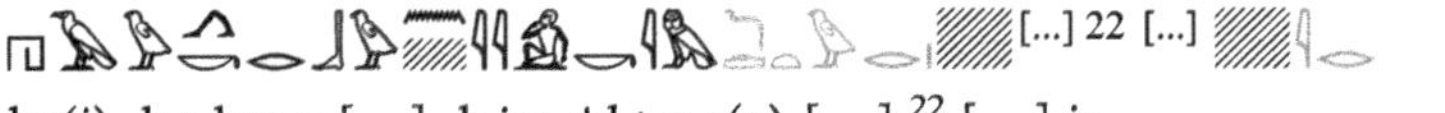

h3(j) m šr.t=s jw=s r ms(j).t jr h3(j) m ḳ3.t=s jw=s r ms(j).t jr

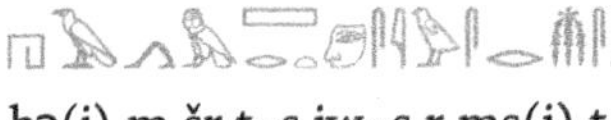

gr.t [...] [23] [...]=s r nḥḥ

Translation

[20] Another time. Oh that calf of Horus! […] [21] that I am with […] Horus and vice-versa. Go down to the place which you […]. The formula to be said is: […] [22] […]. If it comes down from her nostril, she will give birth. However, if it comes down from her vulva, so […] [23] […] she will never (give birth).

No. XXXI

23 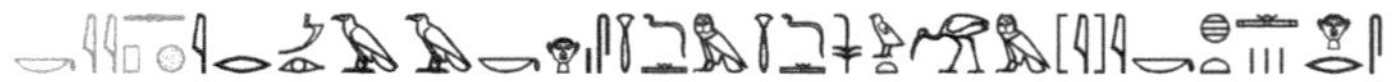

[23] ky-sp jr m33=k ḥr=s w3ḏ m w3ḏ swt gmy=k ḫ.t ḥr=s

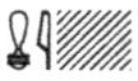 [...] 24 [...] 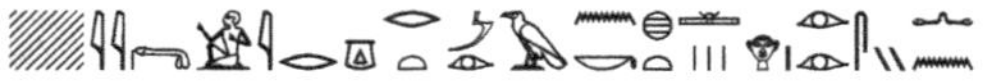

mj […] [24] […]=j jr gr.t m3.n=k ḫ.t ḥr jr.tj=sj nn

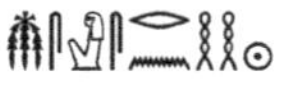

ms(j)=s r nḥḥ

Translation

[23] Another time. If you see her face fresh with brilliance, but find something on her like […] [24] […]. If you find anything on her eyes, she will never give birth

No. XXXII

24 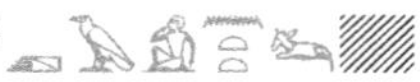 [...] 25 [...] 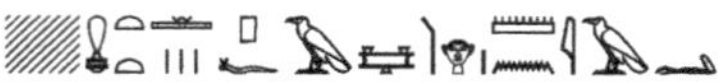

[24] sj3 ntt jw(y.t) […] [25] […] mjtt pf3 ḏbᶜ ḥr mnj3

Translation

[24] Determining the one who will conceive […] [25] […] like that of the finger on the pressure point.

No. XXXIII

25 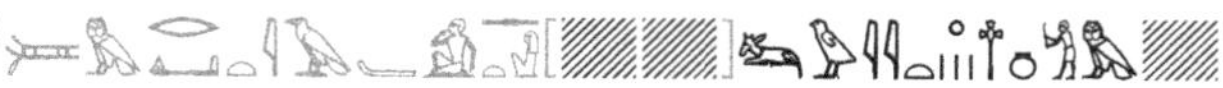 [...] 26 [...]

[25] tm rdj tj3 s.t […] jwy.t nḏ m […] [26] […]

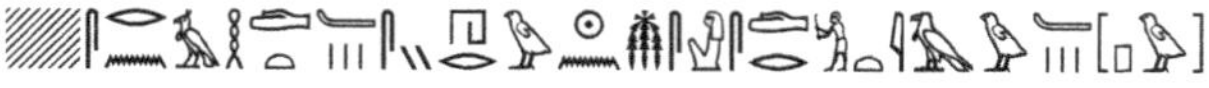

[…]=s r nḥḏ.t=sj hrw n ms(j)=s dr tj3w [pw]

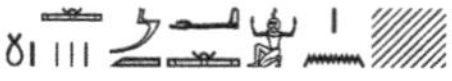 [...]

šs-m3ᶜ ḥḥ n (sp)

Translation

[25] Preventing contractions in the chewing muscles of a woman. […]. Cowpea (*vigna unguiculata*). Grind it with […] [26] […] for her teeth the day she gives birth will drive away the pain on her chewing muscles. This is something really good, (tested) a million (times).

No. XXXIV

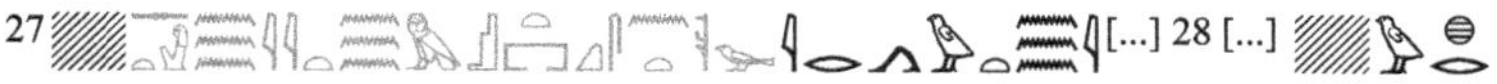

[27] [...] s.t mwy.t m s.t qsn.t jr jw(j).t mwy(.t) j[...] [28] [...].ẖr

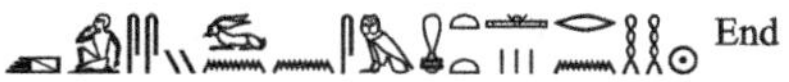

sjꜣ=s sj wnn=s m mtt r nḥḥ

Translation

[27] [...] a woman with local difficulty while urinating. If the urine comes out [...] [28] [...] she observes it, she will be that way for ever.

4. Some final remarks

The ancient Egyptian medical papyri are an important source to understand the Egyptian approach to health treatment. Ancient Egyptian therapeutics were as equally familiar with pharmacy as they were with medicine and incantations. Thanks to the medical papyri, we know details about many of their treatments and prescriptions for diseases. They call for the treatment of many disorders and the use of a variety of substances, plant, animal and mineral.

However, the essential nature of Egyptian healing is deep-seated on religious notions. Hence, magical practices are wholly integrated with empiric-rational approaches to form an integrated but multi-faceted medical therapy.

Traditionally, Egyptology reproduces ideological prejudices regarding the ancient Egyptian medicine empiricism. All supernatural elements are normally treated as mere superstition or, in the best cases, a tool for some placebo effect. On the other hand, though a neurolinguistic approach it becomes clear how intimate was the relation between physical health and spiritual order (in opposition to the cosmic forces of chaos).

One of the main problems on dealing with medical papyri is that they usually do not check or advance with the study of the provided vocabulary. An interesting point for the benefit of Egyptology would be the review of all medical papyri in search of better information about their technical vocabulary, pharmacopoeia, medical substances, and the like.

Such study also considers the proposition of an ontology and semantic analysis. Per definition, ontology, describes the concepts of medical terminologies, practices, and the relation between them, thus, enabling the sharing of medical knowledge. Ontology-based analyses are associated with a tool to represent medical knowledge, thus relying more on the computer science-based understanding of medical terms. This approach is useful for a data entry system, in which the users merely need to browse the hierarchy and select relevant terms.

The language (logos) is the key for a culture's mentality (nous). Thus, it is impossible to deal with language without analysing the thought it's portraying. A Semantic approach aims for the real-world scenario of dealing with grammatically complex terms, which are documented in the ancient Egyptian native language.

The essential nature of Egyptian healing links religious notions and so-called magical practices wholly integrated with empiric-rational approaches to form an integrated but multi-faceted therapeutic.

There are three points to be debated by our source' analysis. Firstly, the usage of a noun, usually translated as "demon", as a synonym for incurable diseases. In case the word is taken literally, then the treatment would be incomplete. Since a "demon" could have been identified and/or exorcized, the therapeutics rather closed the case and move on. Thus, it is most likely the term is here employed as a "harmless" technical term for an untreatable condition.

Secondly, there is a verb, which is synonym with "exorcizing" (evil spirits), although it is here employed in the technical sense of dismissing pain and the expelling of any material residuals from the patient's uterus. By the second time, the term assumes a non-magical usage as a technical jargon. Then, the *materia prima* identifies a magical ingredient: malachite powder. This ingredient would act via the principle of *sympatheia*, as it would restore one's health, thanks to a magical pun (*rebus*) relating malachite, the green colour, and the Egyptian word for "vigor" and "freshness".

Finally, another case shows a fragment of a prayer to Horus in its therapeutics; listed as part of the recommended treatment.

During the preparation of this conclusion, our first impulse was to reduce the words "demon" and "to exorcize" as metaphors, embedded by something as an Ancient Egyptian medical terminology. Then, oppose them to the hymn to Horus and the malachite powder as "magical" elements. However, that would just replicate our prejudice against Egyptian medicine, as we would reproduce the labels of "natural" and "supernatural" as necessary and antagonist categories.

The lack of exorcisms, indexes of demons and magical ingredients (such as amulets) does not "purge" the papyrus from its divine, mythical and magical aspects. The concept of cure is different from the semantic field of the word cure. The cure also performs a transcendent effect, for it changes the patient's destiny. Such effect presupposes some previous formal divine consent.

Therefore, the therapeutics consists of attempts to change the individual destiny. Thus, the transcendent world was unequivocally behind the success or failure of any medical treatment.

Acknowledgements

This book had the support of CHAM (NOVA FCSH/UAc), through the strategic project sponsored by FCT (UIDB/04666/2020).

Further reading

- Frandsen, Paul John. "The Menstrual "Taboo" in Ancient Egypt." Journal of Near Eastern Studies 66, no. 2 (2007): 81 – 106.

- Győry, H. "Interaction of Magic and Science in Ancient Egyptian Medicine" in Zahi Hawass, ed. Egyptology at the Dawn of the Twenty-first Century, Proceedings of the Eighth International Congress of Egyptologists Cairo 2000, Cairo: American University in Cairo Press, 2003, pp. 276 – 83.

- Győry, H. 'Some aspects of magic in ancient Egyptian medicine' in P. Kousoulis (Ed.) Ancient Egyptian Demonology –Studies on the Boundaries between the Demonic and the Divine in Egyptian Magic, Leuven: Peeters, 2011, pp. 151 – 167.

- Johansson, T. The significance of believing in healing – on the therapeutic value of spoken words in ancient Egyptian medical papyri. University essay from Uppsala universitet/Institutionen för arkeologi och antik história, 2019.

- Kousoulis, P. I. M. "Dead entities in living bodies: The demonic influence of the dead in the medical texts" In J.-Cl. Goyon, C. Gardin (Eds.) Proceedings of the Ninth International Congress of Egyptologists – Actes Du Neuvième Congrès International Des Égyptologues. Leuven: Peeters Publishers, 2007, pp. 1043 – 1050.

- Leitz C. P. D.Magical and medical papyri of the New Kingdom. London: British Museum Press for the Trustees of the British Museum, 1999.

- Buchheim, L. "Abortus, Konzeptionsverhütung und Menschwerdung im alten Ägypten" In Deutsche Ärzteblatt–Ärztliche Mitteilungen 61, 45 (1964): 2371 – 2375.

- Haimov-Kochman, R. "Reproduction concepts and practices in ancient Egypt mirrored by modern medicine" in European Journal of Obstetrics and Gynecology and Reproductive Biology, Volume 123, ISSUE 1 (2005): 3 – 8.

- Morice, P.; Josset, P.; Colau, J.-C., "Gynécologie et obstétrique dans l'ancienne Egypte", in Journal de Gynécologie obstétriquee et Biologie de la reproduction, vol.23-2 (1994): 131 – 136.

- Morthon, R.S. "Sexual attitudes, preferences and infections in ancient Egypt" in Genitourin Med. (1995) 71: 180 – 186.

- Nelson, G. S. "Ancient Egyptian obstetrics and gynecology" in Proceedings of the 10th Annual History of Medicine, Calgary: The University of Calgary, 2001.

- O'Dowd, M. J.; Philipp, E. E. The History of Obstetrics and Gynecology. New York: Parthenon Publishing Group, 1994.

- Philippe, M., La gynécologie et l'obstétrique en Egypte pharaonique, thèse de docteur en médecine, Paris V, 1992.

- Richard, M. – C. Pharmacognosie et Traitements Gynecologiques en Egypte Ancienne. Thèse d'Exercice pour le Diplôme d'Etat de Docteur en

Pharmaciesoutenueà l'Université François Rabelais/UFR des Sciences Pharmaceutiques de Tours, 2014.

- Sullivan, R. "Divine and rational: the reproductive health of women in ancient Egypt" in Surv. Obstet. Gynecol. 52 (1997): 635 – 642

- Vernus, P., "Une théorie étiologique de la médecine égyptienne: les souffles vecteurs de maladie, in Revue d'Egyptologie, vol.34 (1982-1983): 121 – 125.

- Von Lieven A.; Quack, J. F. " Ist Liebe eine Frauenkrankheit? Papyrus Berlin P 13602, ein gynäkomagische Handbuch " in Martin, C. J.; Hoogendijk, F. A. J.; van Heel, K. D. Hieratic, Demotic and Greek Studies and Text Editions Of making many Books There is no End: Festschrif in Honour of Sven P Vleeming P.L. Bat 34, Leiden/Boston: Brill, 2018, 257-274.

- Walker, J. "The place of magic in the practice of medicine in ancient Egypt" In Bulletin of the Australian Centre for Egyptology 1 (1990): 85 – 95.

Glossary

Numerals

wꜥ.t – one (feminine)
snw – second
1
2
3
4
ḥḥ - a million

Fractions

gs ½ (half)

Measures

ḥsb – hesb (20, later, 16 hekat)
qd – (¼)3 de hekat = 1/64 hekat
hnw – hin (1/10 hekat)

Generic measurements

bꜣd.t - spoon
mh[r] – jar

ꜣ -

ꜣbd – month
ꜣmmw – anemia
ꜣḥ - porridge
ꜣšr – roast

J –

=j – suffix pronoun: I, my
jꜣb – left hand/side
jꜣr.t – grape
jꜥ(j) – to wash; to clean
jjjw – to leave
jw – Subordination marker
jw(j).t – to come
jwḥ - to hydrate, to wet

jwr(j) – to conceive, to be impregned
jwry.t – beans, cowpea (*vigna unguiculata*)
jwḥw – fruit
jbḥ.w – teeth
jb.t – to be thirsty
jm – there
jmj – together with
jmj.tj – in between (of two referential objects)
.jn – sequential verbal affix: “after x”
jns.t – tight
jr – if, when, in case of
jrj – on that regard, about that, that
jr(j) – to do, to deal, to treat
jr(j) m ẖtjw wʿ.t – to make a sole masse (to mix, to homogenize)
jr.tj – eyes (dual)
jrṯ.t – (cow) milk
jšd – Egyptian balm (*balanites aegyptiaca*)
jd.t - womb

ʿ -

ʿ3 - donkey, ass
ʿ.wt – arms, members, limbs
ʿwy.t – fermented mucilage
ʿmʿm – to lubricate, to rub
mʿ.t – mud
ʿnn – to leave
ʿnnw.t – fruit of the Onenu-tree
ʿntjw – resin of myrrh
ʿq – to enter

W –

w3bw n mn.tj=sj – the root of her tights (perineum?)
w3.t – lateral; side
w3ḏ - green, fresh, vigor, vitality, freshness
w3ḏw – malachite powder
wʿr.tj – legs
wʿḥ - chufa (*cyperus esculentus*)

wpw – to separate
wnm – to eat, to consume
wnn – to exist
wrš – to spend the day
wš – to scratch
wšꜥ - to chew
wšꜥw – to feed, to devour (for animals)
wgp – to smash, to triturate
wḏꜥ - pulp of dates
wḏf – to hesitate, to be late

B –

b3b3.w – cavities
bw – local
bnjw – date syrup
bḥs - calf
bṯw – evil doer (demon); untreatable disease

P –

pw – demonstrative pronoun: this (is); copula particle
pwy – demonstrative pronoun: this (is) vocative
pf – that
pr(j).t – (to) exit
pr[.t]-šnj – white mulberry (*morus alba*)
pḥ(.wj) – tail, back, back side
pḫr – circular
pḫr.t – prescription, medication
ps – to heat, to boil, to cook
psš – to divide
ptr – what (is)

F –

=f – suffix pronoun: he, his
fdq – to sever

M –

m - in, with, as, like, from
m-ḫ.t – after

m-ẖnw – inside

m-gs-ḥr(j) – upside

, m33 -to see

m3w.t – new, recent

mj – like, as

, mjtt, mtt – the same way, similar, likewise, just like that, the same as

mjs.t – liver

mw – water

mwy.t – urine, to urinate

mwy.t m s.t qsn.t – to urinate with local pain or difficulty

mw.t – mother

mw.t-rmṯ - mother of persons (twins?)

mw.t – tuberculum

mn – pain, aching, suffering

mn – to situate

mnj3 - point of pulse

mr – pain

mr.t – to be in love with a bed (to be bedridden)

, mrḥ.t – oil, fat, ointment, unguent

mrḥ.t-m3w.t – new oil

mhwj – rancid oil

mn.t(j) – upper tights

msḥ - crocodile

, ms(j).t – to give birth

ms(j).t(j)=sj – the birth of two children (dual)

ms(j)-t3 - birth-earth (?)

mtjw – tendon, muscle

mdw.t - what is said

N –

n – of (masculine or common); .n - verbal affix (indirect conjugation)

n-mjtt – according to, the same as, like

n(j) – negative particle

n.t – of (feminine)

nw – of (plural)

nw – time, moment

nb – substantive: lord, owner; adjective: all, entire, each, any

nb.t – substantive: lady, owner; adjective: all, entire, each, any

nmsw – effusion

nn – this, those, these

nn – negative particle

nrw – tremor; convulsion

nhq – pain

nḥb.t - throat, neck

nḥd.t – tooth

nqꜥ.wt – ripe figs

nḏm-r(ꜣ) – sweetener of the mouth (breath candy)

ntj – which, that, who (masculine)

ntt - which, that, who (feminine)

nḏ - to grind

nḏm – sweet

nḏr – to press, to force

R –

r – for, to, than

r-nḥḥ - forever, eternally (in negative sentences, never)

r-sꜣ - after

r(ꜣ) – mouth

[...] Fim da coluna 2

rwḏ(.t) – rigid; firm; hard

rḫ[.t] – to know, to be able to

rdj – to give, to allow, to apply (medicine)

rd.wj – feet

H –

hꜣ(j) – to go down, to move, to come

hꜣj – to copulate

hꜣw – to go out

hꜣyw – waves

hrw – day (24 hours)

Ḥ -

ḥꜣtjw – bandages

ḥw(j).t – to be beaten

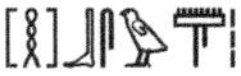

[ḥ]bsw – tissue

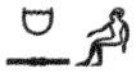

ḥms - to sit

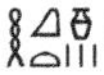

ḥnq.t – beer

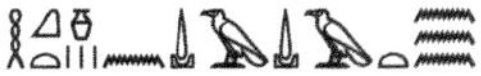

ḥnq.t n ḏ3ḏ3.t – fermented beer

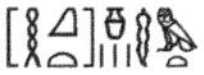

[ḥnq.t]-nḏm.t - sweet beer

ḥn.t-end, extremity, edge

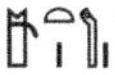

ḥn.t-dbʿ - finger point

Ḥr – Horus

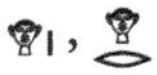

ḥr – on, over, about, that, which, whose

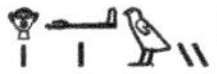

ḥr-ʿ.wj – immediately

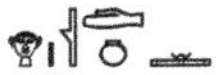

ḥr-qd – completely

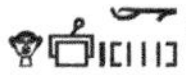

ḥr-s3 - after

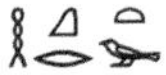

ḥqr.t – fasting

ḥs – excrement

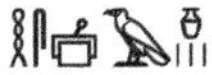

ḥs3 - vegetal mucus

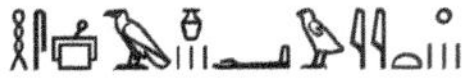

ḥs3-ʿwy.t – fermented vegetal mucus

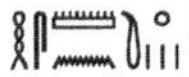

ḥsmn – natron

Ḫ -

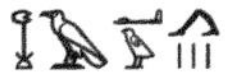

ḫ3ʿw – excretion

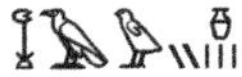

ḫ3wj – emetic

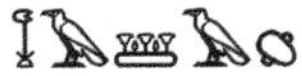

ḫ3š3 - bulging

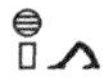

ḫp(j) – to deliver, to menstruate

ḫpr – to manifest

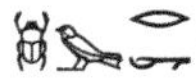

ḫpr-wr – wild carrot (*daucus carota*)

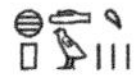

ḫpd.w(j) – buttocks

.ḫr – verbal sequential affix: "and then x"

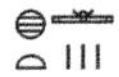

ḫ.t – something, thing.

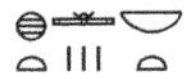

ḫ.t nb.t – anything, everything

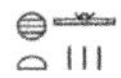

ḫtjw - mass

H̱ –

ẖ3 - to pulverize

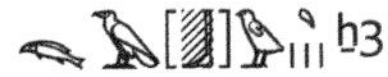

ẖ3[b]w – bellybutton

ẖ.t – belly, body

S –

=s – suffix pronoun: she, her

=sj – suffix pronoun: she, her (dual)

st – it, this, that

sw – he, him

s3ṯw – ground, floor

sj3 - to distinguish, to notice

sjwj – pregnancy

swrj – to drink

swt – in fact, really, after, then

sꜥ3 - to dilatate

sꜥ3m – vitex (*vitex agnus castus*)

sbn.t – to nurse, breastfeeding

sn[ꜥꜥ]w – to reduce, to dilute

snb – health

snb.t – to be healthy

smn – to stabilize

smnḫ - to reduce

, snf - blood

snṯr - incense

srf – to heat, to warm

sḥ3j – to reveal, to expose

, sḥ3w – residual(s)

sḥm – contraceptive

s[ẖ3k]w – to filter

sẖr – to clean, to prepare

ssn.t – to cause an odor

sš – nest

, sqbb – to cool down

s.t - woman

s.t-t3w - woman with fever

s.t - local

s.t-qsn.t – local difficulty

stpw - bandage

[sd]3.t – to move

sḏm.wj - ears

sḏm – to hear, to listen
sḏr.t – to be laying down

Š –

š – fountain
šꜣšꜣ - fruit
š bb – mixed mucilage
šm.t – to walk, to stroll
šfw.t – swollen
šr.t – nostrill, šs-mꜣꜥ - something really good (effective)
šsꜣw – treatment, diagnostic, examine
šsp – palm of hand
šdj – vessel, container
šdj m tkꜣw – burning vessel (brasier, ashtray, incensory)

Q –

qꜣꜥ - vomit
qꜣb.t – breast
qjs (= qꜣs) – to vomit, to puke
qꜥḥw – arching
qmꜣy – to engender, to create
qnqn – to triturate
qsn.t – ill-feeling; difficulty (symptomatic)
qd – to assure; to grant

K –

kꜣp – to fumigate
kꜣ.t – vulva
km.t – illness, disease
knkn – normality, normal estate
kns – groin
ky - (an)other (masculine)
ky-sp - another time
k.t – (an)other (feminine)

G –

[ ] gꜣ.t – privation, deficiency, lacking
gyw – chufa (*cyperus esculentus*)

gm(j) – to find
gnnw – fat from the leg of a goose
grt – in fact, really

T –

t3 - land
t3w – to heat
t3ḫ.t – residual, dregs
tj3w – painful muscular contractions, trismus,
tf3 - that
tm – negative verb (to prevent, not to do)
tḫb – wet, soggy

Ṯ -

ṯ3 - bulb
ṯ3 n ḥḏw – onion bulb
ṯnw – each (each time x happens ... then each time y results)
ṯs-pḫr(w) – vice-versa (circular link)

D –

dw3.t – early morning
dwn – to stand
dr – to keep away, to exorcise, to expel
dq3 (= dqr) – fruit
d.t – hand

Ḏ -

ḏ3y(.t) – wound
ḏ3dy.t – fermented/burning beer
ḏ3ḏ3w – special pot to prepare medicines
ḏ3ḏ3.t – around
ḏbꜥ - finger
ḏ3ḏ3 - top, head
ḏd - to say, to tell

Author details

Helena Trindade Lopes[1]* and Ronaldo G. Gurgel Pereira[2]

1 Nova Faculdade de Ciências Sociais e Humanas, FCSH, Universidade NOVA de Lisboa/CHAM - CHAM, Faculdade de Ciências Sociais e Humanas, FCSH, Universidade NOVA de Lisboa, Lisboa, Portugal

2 CHAM, Faculdade de Ciências Sociais e Humanas, FCSH, Universidade NOVA de Lisboa, Lisboa, Portugal

*Address all correspondence to: mh.lopes@fcsh.unl.pt

References

[1] Nunn, J. F. *Ancient Egyptian Medicine*. London: British Museum Press, 1996.

[2] Griffith, F. Ll. *The Petrie Papyri: Hieratic Papyri from Kahun and Gurob*. London: Bernard Quaritch, 1898, pp. 5-11; pl. V-VI.

[3] Guermeur, I. "Entre magie et médecine. L'exemple du papyrus Brooklyn 47.218.2", Égypte, Afrique et Orient 71 (2013), pp. 11 – 22.

[4] Grapow, H. *et al. Grundriss der Medizin der alten Aegypter*, 9 vols, Berlin: Akademie-Verlag, 1954-1973.

[5] Stevens, J. M. "Gynaecology from ancient Egypt: the papyrus Kahun. A translation of the oldest treatise on gynaecology that has survived from the ancient world" in *Medical Journal of Australia,* 2(25–26), 949–952, 1975.

[6] Bardinet, Th. *Les Papyrus médicaux de l'Égypte pharaonique*, Paris: Fayard, 1995.

[7] Quirke, S. *Digital Egypt for Universities. Manuscript for the health of mother and child (Kahun Medical Papyrus UC 32057)*. 2002. http://www.digitalegypt.ucl.ac.uk/med/birthpapyrus.html [2020-06-05].

[8] Collier, M.; Quirke, S. *The UCL Lahun Papyri: Religious, Literary, Legal, Mathematical and Medical*. Oxford: Archeopress, 2004.

[9] Fournier, D. *Le papyrus gynécologique de Kahun (Petrie Museum of Egyptian Archaeology, University College London, UC 32057). Transcription-Translittération-Traduction. Considérations lexicales, syntaxiques, sémantiques, commentaires médicaux.* Paris: Éditions PAM, 2017.

[10] Leake, Ch. D. *The Old Egyptian Medical Papyri* (= Logan Clendening Lectures on the History and Philosophy of Medicine, 2. Serie). Lawrence, Kansas: University of Kansas Press, 1952.

[11] Reeves C. *Egyptian Medicine*. London: Shire Publications, 1992.

[12] Stegbauer, K. *Magie als Waffe gegen Schlangen in der ägyptischen Bronzezeit*. Ägyptologische Studien Leipzig, 1, 2019.

[13] Strouhal, E., Vachala; B., Vymazalová; H. *Medicine of the Ancient Egyptians: 1: Surgery, , Obstetrics, and Pediatrics*. Cairo: American University in Cairo Press, 2014.

[14] Pereira, R. G. G. *Gramática Fundamental de Egípcio Hieroglífico*. Lisboa: Chiado, 2016.

[15] Pommenering, T. "Die SsAw-Lehrtexte der heilkundlichen Literatur des Alten Ägypten. Texttraditionen und Textgeschichte." In: D. Bawanypcck, A. Imhausen (Eds). *Traditions of Written Knowledge in Ancient Egypt and Mesopotamia. Proceedings of two Workshops held at Goethe-University, Frankfurt/Main, in December 2001 and May 2012.* Alter Orient und Altes Testament, 403, Münster: Ugarit Verlag, 2014, pp. 7-47.

[16] Hannig, R. *Grosses Handwörterbuch Ägyptisch-Deutsch*. Mainz: Philipp von Zabern, 2006.

[17] Smith, L. "The Kahun Gynaecological Papyrus: Ancient Egyptian medicine" in *Journal of Family Planning and Reproductive Health Care* 37(1):54–5, 2011.

[18] Rouffet, F. "Les ingrédients dans les prescriptions médico-magiques égyptiennes" in Égypte, Afrique et Orient 71, (2013), pp. 23 – 32.

[19] Nunn, J. F. "Disease" in *The Oxford Encyclopedia of Ancient Egypt* (dir. D. B.

Redford), vol. 3, Cairo: The American University in Cairo Press. 2001, pp. 396-401.

[20] Verkaik, S., Kamperman, A. M., van Westrhenen, R., Schulte, P. F. "The treatment of premenstrual syndrome with preparations of *Vitex agnus castus*: a systematic review and meta-analysis". American Journal of Obstetrics and Gynecology. 217 (2): 150–166, 2017.

[21] Wang, C. P., Wang Y., Wang, X., Zhang, X., Ye, J. F., Hu, L. S., Kong, L. D. "Mulberroside a possesses potent uricosuric and nephroprotective effects in hyperuricemic mice". *Planta Medica*, 10 Dec 2010, 77(8): 786 – 794.

[22] Daya L., Chothani, H. U."A review on *Balanites aegyptiaca* Del (desert date): phytochemical constituents, traditional uses, and pharmacological activity". Pharmacognosy Reviews. 5 (9): 55–62, 2011.

[23] Iwu, M. M. *Handbook of African medicinal plants.* Boca Raton: CRC Press, 1993.

[24] Vernus, P. "Le rébus dans l'écriture hiéroglyphique de l'Égypte pharaonique: un procédé cognitif" in: C.-A. Brisset *et al.* (Eds.) Rébus d'ici et d'ailleurs: écriture, image, signe. Paris: Hemisphères, 2018, pp. 45 – 65.

www.ingramcontent.com/pod-product-compliance
Lightning Source LLC
Chambersburg PA
CBHW081246190326
41458CB00016B/5938